ARE YOUR
MEDS MAKING
YOU SICK?

Ordering

Trade bookstores in the U.S. and Canada please contact:

Publishers Group West
1700 Fourth Street, Berkeley CA 94710
Phone: (800) 788-3123   Fax: (800) 351-5073

Hunter House books are available at bulk discounts for textbook course adoptions;
to qualifying community, health-care, and government organizations; and
for special promotions and fund-raising. For details please contact:

Special Sales Department
Hunter House Inc., PO Box 2914, Alameda CA 94501-0914
Phone: (510) 865-5282   Fax: (510) 865-4295
E-mail: ordering@hunterhouse.com

Individuals can order our books from most bookstores,
by calling **(800) 266-5592**, or from our website at
www.hunterhouse.com

ARE YOUR MEDS MAKING YOU SICK?

A Pharmacist's Guide to
Avoiding Dangerous Drug Interactions,
Reactions and Side Effects

ROBERT STEVEN GOLD, RPH, MBA

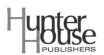

Copyright © 2011 by Robert Gold

Hunter House Inc., Publishers
PO Box 2914
Alameda CA 94501-0914

Library of Congress Cataloging-in-Publication Data
Gold, Robert Steven
Are your meds making you sick? : a pharmacist's guide to avoiding dangerous drug interactions, reactions, and side-effects / Robert Steven Gold.
      p.   cm.
Includes bibliographical references and index.
ISBN 978-0-89793-570-8 (pbk.)
1. Drugs — Side effects — Handbooks, manuals, etc.   I. Title.
RM302.5.G65 2011
615.7'042 — dc23   2011023472

Project Credits

Cover Design: Brian Dittmar Design, Inc.   Interns: Jack Duffy and Erica M. Lee
Book Production: John McKercher   Publicity & Marketing: Sean Harvey
Proofreader: John David Marion   Rights Coordinator: Candace Groskreutz
Indexer: Candace Hyatt   Order Fulfillment: Washul Lakdhon
Managing Editor: Alexandra Mummery   Administrator: Theresa Nelson
Acquisitions Assistant: Elizabeth Kracht   Computer Support: Peter Eichelberger
Developmental Editors: Kelsey Comes and Mary Claire Blakeman
Copy Editors: Mary Miller and Heather Wilcox
Senior Marketing Associate: Reina Santana
Customer Service Manager: Christina Sverdrup
Publisher: Kiran S. Rana

Printed and bound by Bang Printing, Brainerd, Minnesota
Manufactured in the United States of America

9 8 7 6 5 4 3 2 1   First Edition   11 12 13 14 15

Contents

Introduction 1
    Worse Than We Know. 2
    Guidelines Needed. 5
    Report Problems. 6
    Be Proactive. 8

How to Use This Book 9
    Medication-Induced Mysteries 9
    Trail of Clues: Where to Find Information
    on Your Medications in this Book 11

1 The Sixteen Rules of Safe Medication Use 13
    Protect Yourself: Record and Report 23

**2 Are Your Meds Causing Problems in
the Lungs or Heart?** 24
    Medication-Induced Lung Disease. 24
    Medication-Induced Pneumonia 31
    Medication-Induced Respiratory Insufficiency
    (Breathing Problems) 37
    Medication-Induced Cough 44
    Medication-Induced Arrhythmia. 50

**3 Are Your Meds Causing Kidney, Calcium, Liver, Pancreas,
or Diabetic Complications?** 58
    Medication-Induced Renal (Kidney) Failure 58
    Medication-Induced Hypercalcemia
    (Excessive Calcium) 66
    Medication-Induced Liver Dysfunction 72

Medication-Induced Pancreatitis 79
Medication-Induced Diabetic Complications 84

4 Are Your Meds Playing Tricks with Your Mind? 91
Medication-Induced Psychosis — Case 1 91
Medication-Induced Psychosis — Case 2 98
Medication-Induced Falling 103
Medication-Induced Serotonin Syndrome 109
Medication-Induced Seizure 116
Medication-Induced Digoxin Toxicity
in Heart Patients 123
Medication-Induced Hearing Loss 130

5 Are Your Meds Causing Bleeding Problems? 136
Medication-Induced Subcutaneous
Bleeding (Bruising) 136
Medication-Induced Upper-GI Bleeding 145
Medication-Induced Gastrointestinal Ulceration 151

**6 Are Your Meds Causing Strange and
Unusual Symptoms?** 160
Medication-Induced Intestinal Blockage 160
Medication-Induced Lactic Acidosis 167
Medication-Induced Hypoglycemia
(Low Blood Sugar) 174
Medication-Induced Stevens-Johnson Syndrome
(a Painful Rash That Spreads and Blisters Like a Burn) 181
Medication-Induced Rhabdomyolysis (Muscle Pain) . 189
Medication-Induced Hyperkalemia
(High Blood Potassium Levels) 198
Medication-Induced Diarrhea 204
Medication-Induced Movement Disorder 210
Medication-Induced Problems from
Lack of Oversight 217
Opiate Withdrawal 224

Conclusion 231

Appendix: Reader's Guide to Medications 232

Notes 235

Glossary 259

Important Web Resources 267

My Medicine Record 268

Index 270

Important Note

The material in this book is intended to provide a review of resources and information related to adverse drug reactions as seen by a hospital pharmacist. Every effort has been made to provide accurate and dependable information. However, professionals in the field may have differing opinions, and change is always taking place. Any of the treatments described herein should be undertaken only under the guidance of a licensed health-care practitioner. The author, editors, and publishers cannot be held responsible for any error, omission, professional disagreement, outdated material, or adverse outcomes that derive from use of any of these treatments or information resources in this book, either in a program of self-care or under the care of a licensed practitioner.

Please note: Any similarities between these cases and actual people are purely coincidental. The patient cases are based on actual drugs but do not portray any specific patient seen by the author. Always check with your physician before changing therapies. Throughout the text, the most recent statistics available are provided. It is rare that large scale studies are done regularly on many of these drugs, thus *Are Your Meds Making You Sick?* relies on the seminal or most influential studies, some of which may be over five years old.

Introduction

Did you know that an adverse drug reaction could pose more danger to your life than a car crash? In fact, according to the Food and Drug Administration (FDA), these harmful reactions to medications cause more deaths annually than all motor vehicle accidents, homicides, and airplane crashes combined!

Specifically, the FDA estimates that 100,000 people are killed by drug reactions per year.[1] That number echoes the results of a study published in the *Journal of the American Medical Association* that stated that an estimated 100,000 deaths occur yearly in the United States as a result of and in association with adverse drug reactions. This same article also reported that adverse drug reactions resulted in 700,000 hospital emergency-room visits in 1994.[2]

Another source pegs the enormous number of serious injuries caused by adverse drug reactions at 2.1 million. Economically speaking, these incidents are responsible for an estimated 1.56 to 4 billion dollars in health-care costs annually.[3] Put in perspective, adverse drug reactions could be the fourth-leading cause of death in the United States, placing them ahead of pulmonary disease, AIDS, diabetes, pneumonia, and kidney failure.[4]

With the patient population in today's health-care system living longer and, therefore, likely to be on more medications, adverse drug reaction rates are anticipated to continue to climb. Consider these facts:

- Between 1998 and 2005 the number of adverse drug reactions and subsequent deaths due to these reactions increased by a factor of nearly 2.6![5]

- In another study based on analysis of 50 million U.S. death certificates, 12,426 deaths in 2004 were caused from medication mistakes at home. This statistic represents an increase of more than 700 percent since 1983.[6]

Worse Than We Know...

As startling as these statistics are, the problem may be even worse than most people realize. According to the FDA, fewer than *1 percent* of all adverse drug reactions are reported. This information is quite troubling for the consumer. If fewer than 1 percent of all adverse reactions are reported, the problems that are now becoming apparent may be grossly underrepresented.[7]

For the record, according to the FDA, a serious adverse drug reaction is one in which "the patient outcome is death, life threatening (real risk of dying), hospitalization (initial or prolonged), disability (significant, persistent, or permanent), congenital anomaly, or required intervention to prevent permanent impairment or damage." All these reactions are serious problems, but the most alarming aspect is that many of these reactions can be avoided.[8]

In a perfect health-care system, your dispensing pharmacist would have access to your medical history and current records, including kidney and liver lab values. (Note: The term "lab values" is explained further in Chapter 1, as well as in the Glossary.) The pharmacist would be able to meet with you and to review all your medications to ensure safety, and then they would counsel you regarding the adverse side effects associated with your medications. The pharmacist would also have the information needed to make recommendations on alterations in therapy and lab test monitoring. The system would track what the hospitals and doctors have recorded, and this information would be made available to you. If you experienced any health changes, the system would update your records and alert health-care professionals to make sure you are not at risk. Unfortunately, this system is not in place today.

The Case That Started It All

One afternoon as I arrived at the hospital where I worked as a pharmacist, I noticed Joe outside having a cigarette break. I

(cont'd.)

half-jokingly suggested that he quit smoking; he laughed it off, asking what good it would it do him now.

You see, Joe, only 58-years-old, was in the final stages of lung cancer. He had been admitted to the hospital for palliative care; that is, for a pain management regimen that was designed to make Joe's life a little easier to bear in his last few months.

As part of his treatment for lung cancer, Joe had undergone multiple rounds of radiation and chemotherapy. He had received cisplatin, a chemotherapy drug commonly used with lung cancer patients—and a drug that is notoriously hard on the kidneys. The cisplatin had caused significant damage to Joe's kidneys and, as a result, they were unable to filter or remove certain medications from his system.

I had been following Joe's condition for a few days because, during the course of my work in the pharmacy, I noticed he was receiving meperidine intravenously. Meperidine is a pain killer that some people may recognize more easily by its trade name, Demerol. At the dose Joe was receiving—25 mg per hour—neurological side effects become more prominent, including dizziness, sedation, and, more seriously, seizures. Another side effect Joe experienced was kidney failure, presumably due to the kidney-damaging impact of his chemotherapy treatment with cisplatin. When meperidine is metabolized, or cleared from the body, it transforms into an active metabolite called normeperidine. Because of the damage from the cisplatin, however, Joe's kidneys were unable to remove the meperidine from his system.

Knowing the side effects of both the meperidine (Demerol) as well as the cisplatin, I informed Joe that he could end up having a seizure, because his kidneys weren't functioning as they should. I suggested that he try morphine instead. Morphine, which works just as well for pain, does not have a history of causing seizures and does not require dose adjustment for kidney problems. Joe said that he was happy with his meperidine because it was controlling his pain, so he would rather leave it alone.

I then followed up with his physician. Joe's doctor stated that if the meperidine was controlling Joe's pain, then it was fine. I pointed out that with the high dose of meperidine and

(cont'd.)

Joe's kidney damage, he might experience seizures due to his kidneys' inability to remove the active metabolite, but the doctor chose to ignore the warning.

Over time, the meperidine built up in Joe's body, and a seizure occurred on a Friday. The following Monday, when I returned to the hospital, I stopped in to check on Joe. I asked him how he was doing, and unfortunately, he confirmed my prediction, telling me he had experienced a horrible seizure a couple days earlier. I then learned that his physician had decided to switch Joe to morphine, and Joe did not experience another seizure during his final months of life.

That experience with Joe dramatically demonstrated to me the consequences of adverse drug reactions and made me even more aware of the recurring problems with certain medications that I was noticing as part of my job in the pharmacy. So after witnessing what happened to Joe, I began collecting data on these problems.

This research served me well when my own father also experienced a negative side effect from one of the drugs he was taking. I was able to quickly recognize that my Dad's problem was medication related, and I was also able to intervene and have his prescription changed to a drug with less-harmful side effects.

Although I've had five years of pharmacy school and more than twenty years of experience, I realized that people without a medical background just do not have the experience and the knowledge to identify common drug-induced illnesses. They cannot care for themselves or a loved one as I could my father. And thus the idea for writing *Are Your Meds Making You Sick?* was born. Through my research, I found that the problems I was witnessing at our hospital in Indiana were the same ones being seen all over the nation. According to an article published in the *Journal of the American Medical Association* in October 2006,[9] adverse reactions from prescription medications cause more than seven hundred thousand trips to emergency rooms each year. I don't know about you, but I certainly don't want myself or anyone I care about to be among those seven hundred thousand. And no one wants to be among the estimated 100,000 people who die every year from these reactions. Be-

(cont'd.)

cause of these sobering statistics, my main goal for this book is to make the public aware of common signs and symptoms of adverse drug reactions, what to do if they experience them, and how to prevent them from occurring.

Certainly, I am not alone in pursuing this goal. For instance, the Joint Commission (previously called The Joint Commission on the Accreditation of Health Care) promotes National Patient Safety Goals that include recommendations for preventing medication-induced problems. Notably, since 2001 the Commission no longer recommends using meperidine (Demerol). The drug has since been removed from many hospital formularies because of the increased risk of seizures and other problems that occur when the drug is used for elderly patients. That recommendation came too late to help a patient like Joe, but it is an example of a step in the right direction. Much more needs to be done—and one of the best things you can do is to educate yourself on this issue. I encourage you to read the Introduction to *Are Your Meds Making You Sick?* and also the section on "How to Use This Book" so you will understand the concept and style of the book. I hope you enjoy reading it, but, more importantly, I hope you learn from it and glean life-saving information.

Guidelines Needed...

It is true that drug manufacturers supply official FDA-approved information guides for prescribing medications. Guides are also available in books, studies, databases, and government guidelines for nursing homes. Despite all this information, however, the rules are not being followed. People are still being prescribed drugs that should be avoided given their specific health conditions or are being placed on doses that are too high for them. An optimal therapeutic regimen for individuals should include having a pharmacist or a doctor review their medications and lab tests to make sure their drugs are providing the best results possible. But this is not always the case.

What is needed is a mandated set of guidelines that would provide medical professionals with information pertaining to inappropriate medications for certain populations. These guidelines would include a dosing range appropriate for patients according to their ages, weights, and kidney/liver functions, and they would make lab reports available to pharmacists to review so appropriate dosages could be evaluated. Although that perfect system is not available to everyone, *Are Your Meds Making You Sick?* attempts to bring that perfect system closer to reality by informing you of what to watch for and what to do to prevent the most common adverse events from happening.

When you are admitted to the hospital, most of the time a hospitalist is going to care for you. A "hospitalist," as the name implies, is a general physician who only treats patients who are admitted to the hospital. They may prescribe new medications for you or send you home with new medications. Additionally, because of cost considerations, hospitals sometimes substitute new medications for other drugs you may have been taking prior to hospitalization. The problem with these procedures is that a hospitalist is not your family doctor. This person often doesn't know what medications you were on previously and may inadvertently prescribe duplicate medications. Some of the substitutions may have different side effects or interactions with other medications. The hospitalist also does not necessarily communicate directly with your family doctor, which can lead to serious problems with your mix of medications. Ask the hospitalist about any changes they make to your drug regimen, and tell your family doctor about them to determine which medications your doctor would like you to continue — or discontinue.

Report Problems...

As a consumer, it is of the utmost importance that you report any problems you notice once you start taking a medication. Report them to your physician or pharmacist so the FDA is aware of the side effects you may be experiencing with your new medication.

You, as the patient, would be the first to notice any unusual signs and symptoms that might arise, so if something does not seem right after starting a new medication, talk to your doctor or pharmacist as soon as possible.

As new drugs are introduced into the market, drug companies urge physicians to prescribe them. Your doctor weighs the risks along with the possible benefits of a new treatment when making a decision on your drug therapy. Some clinical trials may include only six hundred to one thousand patients before the FDA approves the drug. However, many serious adverse drug reactions are rare, so they may not be noticed in the clinical trials. The FDA requires manufacturers to monitor a drug after it is placed on the market, which is called postmarketing surveillance or Phase IV testing. The postmarketing surveillance usually lasts approximately eighteen months. During this time, patients, doctors, and pharmacists are urged to report any side effects and serious problems noticed with the new medication to the drug company. This monitoring helps ensure that the medication is safe and that no serious rare adverse reactions are occurring with widespread use of the medication.

The problem is that postmarketing surveillance does not *require* reporting. No one, including doctors or pharmacists, has to report any adverse reaction a patient may experience from a drug. Herein lies the problem with the FDA's surveillance system: It relies heavily on outside observation and voluntary reporting to catch many of the rare adverse reactions that patients may experience; therefore, many critics believe the FDA is missing numerous serious adverse events. For example, a medication that causes 1 in 3,000 patients to have liver failure may not be noticed until the drug is on the market. This widespread use allows the FDA and the drug company to catch any major problems with its medication, but after the drug has been prescribed to 300,000 patients, 100 of them could possibly have life-threatening liver failure. That is a significant number of patients.

As a consumer, you may also report any problems you believe to be associated with your medications via the FDA's MedWatch

website at http://www.fda.gov/medwatch/report/consumer/con
sumer.htm.

Be Proactive...

As a responsible patient, be proactive with your medications. Discuss the risks of taking the medication with your doctor and pharmacist. Know the possible and likely side effects, minor and serious,
so you can recognize any problems before it becomes too late, and
don't rely solely on advertisements to tell you what those possible
side effects are!

Prevention is the key to protecting yourself. Recently, weather
radios have become highly sought after as a means of protection
from the dangers of severe weather, such as tornadoes. It is interesting to note that during 2007 only 81 deaths were attributed to tornadoes, yet thousands of Americans looking to protect themselves and
their family from storms purchased weather radios.[10] You should
realize that by taking a few simple steps outlined in this book, you
may be able to prevent much more common tragedies. This book
provides the tools necessary to recognize major drug interactions
and adverse effects so you can protect yourself from the dangers of
too many medications.

This book presents many case examples so that you, the consumer, will be better prepared to notice and to prevent such adverse
reactions. Many commonly prescribed drugs on the market can be
dangerous when given to the wrong patient and can have serious
life-threatening side effects. On a daily basis, patients are admitted
to hospitals because of adverse drug reactions that can and should
have been prevented with proper precautions during their prior
treatment. It is up to you as the patient to be aware and informed
to prevent these errors from happening. I see it as a challenge and a
responsibility to educate the consumer about the dangers of some
medications. I want to train the public to think like a pharmacist,
always being aware of the possible dangers that go along with the
benefits of prescription and nonprescription drugs.

How to Use This Book

I feel strongly that everyone learns more when they're having a little fun. Therefore, I wrote each chapter in this book (after Chapter 1) as a series of mini-mysteries in which you are asked to solve a "case" and identify the cause of adverse drug reactions triggered by various medications. Each scenario illustrates a particular medication-induced problem, and similar health issues are grouped together by chapter.

You may want to read through these cases as you would a detective novel. Or, alternatively, you can look up the medication or medical condition that is of particular concern to you in a special Index in the Appendix which is described in the section below entitled, "Trail of Clues: Where to Find Information on Your Medications in this Book."

But first, take a look at the following overview to get an idea of how each case is set up within the chapters. (Note: Some of the technical aspects related to the lab readings and dosages that are referenced throughout the book are defined in the Glossary.)

Medication-Induced Mysteries

When you read about the experiences of other people, it makes it easier to understand how your meds could be making you sick. Information on these patient experiences are broken down into the following categories for each case in this book:

THE PATIENT

A quick description of the patient, their disease status, and other tidbits of information that may help you solve the "mystery" surrounding an adverse drug reaction.

THE SYMPTOMS

What goes wrong and what the patient feels.

THE SUSPECTS

A list and description of all the patient's medications.

LET'S RECAP

After each patient's situation is described, a recap is presented in the Summary Report.

SUMMARY REPORT

This section provides critical details including assessments of the patient's medications, their doses and frequencies, and any laboratory or X-ray findings.

SOLVE THE MYSTERY

Can you find the answer to the mystery before it is provided for you?

The Culprit

Identifies the "culprit drug," including why and how it causes problems for the patient.

The Accomplice

A description of any other medications, lifestyle choices, or factors that have been making the problem worse.

THE SOLUTION

What the doctors and pharmacists did to help the patient.

WHAT ARE YOUR CHANCES?

An estimate of the annual incidence of adverse events associated with the "culprit" medication(s).

(Note: Throughout each discussion in the "What Are Your Chances?" sections, I attempt to make educated guesses regarding the incidence I believe to be occurring on an annual basis. These estimates are based on the recent year's prescription data paired with the patient population and the estimated incidence according to the package inserts for the medications. I did not conduct clinical trials investigating the incidence; these are purely my best intelligent guesses about the frequency of incidence for these adverse events. This section also contains data from the website https://www .prosoftedc.com/aers.html, which draws information from the FDA Adverse Event Reporting System that doctors and other health-care professionals use to document the adverse reactions to drugs. The website provides access to incidence reporting but is a little technical, so I pulled out the pertinent information to add to each chapter. Access the website yourself, or just check out this section in every chapter. Be advised that using the website to locate the exact information you are looking for is not an easy task. In fact, the FDA publishes the data once every quarter on its website and leaves the data in a form that only a computer whiz would be able to interpret. This website takes the obscure data from the FDA and attempts to present it in a readable format. It is still very difficult to find precisely what you need, but it is better than nothing.)

 HELPFUL ADVICE

Helpful advice to prevent an adverse drug reaction closes out each "case" in the book.

Trail of Clues: Where to Find Information on Your Medications in this Book

To make it easier for you to find out about possible problems with a medication used by you (or a loved one), a special Index has been created, and you will find it on page 232. One medication may be prescribed to patients with a variety of conditions, or a medication may produce a variety of side effects. That is why certain drugs are discussed in more than one chapter. To locate the drug that matches your health problem, look for the name of the medication in the left-most column of the alphabetical list in the special index. Then follow it across the columns to pinpoint the medical condition or symptom that concerns you most. The section of the special index shown below gives you an example of how to find information on a drug like acetaminophen, which may be a "suspect" in several scenarios in the book.

READER'S GUIDE TO MEDICATIONS

Medication	Body Area	Medical Condition/ Symptom	Chapter
Acetaminophen	Liver	Nausea, weakness	3, Medication-Induced Liver Dysfunction

CHAPTER 1

The Sixteen Rules of Safe Medication Use

Based on the my work in a hospital setting I have found there are sixteen rules to keep in mind if you are trying to determine if your meds are making you sick.

1. Learn Which Medications Are Causing People to Be Admitted to Emergency Rooms

Because adverse drug reactions are woefully underreported, many people are unaware of problems with their medications until they land in the emergency room (ER). Statistics from ERs, then, can give us a snapshot of what is actually happening to thousands of patients whose medications have made them sick. Based on figures from emergency-room visits across the United States, several medications have been found to be the most troublesome — in particular, insulin, digoxin, and warfarin. Although other prescription drugs can cause some severe reactions, these three drugs can set off a rapid series of negative events with no warning, and using them increases your risk of medication-induced disease. Results of reports to the Food and Drug Administration (FDA) regarding adverse drug effects were published in the *Archives of Internal Medicine,* and these results showed insulin to be the second-most-dangerous medication leading to disabilities or serious outcomes, with warfarin being rated close behind as number seven. Acetaminophen (Tylenol) was rated fifth on the list of medications most commonly identified as causing adverse drug reactions such as liver failure.[1] (This does not, however, suggest that you should change your regimen on your own—see Rule #5 on page 16). By paying attention to these results as well as the emergency-room statistics (which are mentioned throughout this book), you will improve your chances of avoiding dangerous reactions to your medications.

2. Know Your Kidney Lab Values

Health-care professionals may use the term "lab values" to describe the numerical value of certain lab-test results. You may also hear the term "reference range" used for this purpose, because lab values usually represent a *range* of numbers that emerge after testing a large group of people to establish a baseline for "normal" functioning. But the word "normal" can be misleading, because a test result that could be "normal" for a fifty-year-old may not necessarily be "normal" for an eighty-year-old. Therefore, instead of discussing test results as being "normal" or "abnormal," doctors, pharmacists, and others in the medical field look at the lab values or reference ranges to determine whether your results present a cause for concern or not.

All of this information from your tests becomes particularly important in assessing your kidney function and your risk of adverse drug reactions because of a simple fact: Many medicines are removed from the body through the kidneys. When this filtration system does not work as it should, a drug remains in the body for a longer period of time, which then increases the likelihood of problematic reactions. Luckily, simple blood tests can quickly evaluate a person's kidney function. These tests include those that check your levels of serum creatinine (SCr) and blood urea nitrogen (BUN). Knowing the critical lab values from these tests can help your doctor determine what dose or which drug to select to keep you safe, especially because there are several medications that should *not* be prescribed when your kidney function is below par. If you are at home and begin to notice a decrease in your urine output, it could be a sign of declining kidney function. Contact your physician before taking your medications, because serious consequences could result if you ignore this condition. Recognizing whether your kidneys are working properly or not, and discussing their function with your doctor and pharmacist can help prevent adverse reactions. The current health-care system does not adequately catch medications that should be avoided when a patient has reduced kidney function. Therefore, be aware of your kidney lab values, and stay in communication with your pharmacist and doctor if you notice any changes. (For further information, you can also read the section on "Understanding Your Lab Values" on the website of the National Kidney Foundation, www.kidney.org.)

3. Know Your Liver Lab Values

Like your kidneys, your liver also removes many drugs from your body, causing similar problems to those of kidney malfunction when the organ is impaired. Again, simple lab tests—including those for checking your levels of alanine transaminase (ALT), aspartate aminotransferase (AST), albumin, alkaline phosphatase (Alk Phos), and bilirubin—can detect how well your liver is functioning. Knowing your lab values for the above liver-function tests, as well as which drugs can damage your liver, empowers you to understand your medications and possibly avoid adverse reactions. For example, drinking alcohol can damage your liver and change the way it clears some drugs from your system. Taking acetaminophen and drinking alcohol at the same time can cause changes in your metabolism and increase the risk of liver toxicity—clearly a situation to avoid if you want to stay healthy.

4. Be Aware That Elderly Patients Are Different from Younger People

Elderly patients, generally speaking, react differently to the same medications that younger adults can tolerate well, and they are more likely to experience severe reactions. Many physical parameters in the elderly body, such as drug excretion, metabolism, body weight, cognitive function, and general health, change over time. Elderly patients should be monitored more closely than younger patients who are taking the same medication. A good reference book for older adult doses is *Lexi-Comp's Geriatric Dosage Handbook*. The book covers many useful topics pertaining to drugs, such as warnings, adverse reactions, drug interactions, monitoring parameters, dosing for elderly patients, and special geriatric considerations.

5. Take Your Medications as Your Doctor Prescribed

Taking your drugs as prescribed by your doctor protects you in several ways. First, the doctor chooses a dose with a set frequency for your condition. The pharmacist then evaluates what the doctor has directed you to do and dispenses the medication in line with these directions. Although errors can occur during this process, you are far safer if you follow the prescribed guidelines. Dosing yourself based on the way you feel on a certain day could have severe effects. *Always* keep your physician honestly informed if you decide to take a different dosage from that which you have been prescribed (or, preferably, talk to your doctor *before* you make any self-determined changes).

6. Know Your Lab-Test Schedule

The dosage adjustment of many medications is based on lab values that must be obtained from regularly scheduled tests. As explained previously, your kidney and liver functions are evaluated based on blood tests. These tests can help a physician determine the drugs and dosage levels that are appropriate for you. Missing these scheduled lab tests can lead to your receiving the wrong dosage as your health conditions change, and that can cause additional problems or may even result in your hospitalization.

7. Know Your Medication's Monitoring Parameters

The term "monitoring parameters" is one that pharmacists and others in the medical profession use when they are talking about the effectiveness of a prescription medication. In other words, these parameters serve as guidelines that can show if a certain drug is working or not. For example, medications for high blood pressure can be evaluated for effectiveness if a doctor measures a patient's blood pressure rate at regular intervals. Some medications can also be evaluated at home. Patients and caregivers should talk with physicians (or pharmacists) about how to monitor these medications to help avoid the use of certain drugs when readings are outside of given parameters.

8. Do Not Hesitate to Call Your Doctor

If you become ill with a viral or bacterial infection or another illness that changes aspects of your behavior, such as decreased fluid intake, vomiting, or diarrhea, it may not seem life-threatening. When you are taking medications, however, an illness, or even a discomforting condition like diarrhea, can have more serious implications. Do not wait to contact your physician if you become ill, and be sure to ask specific questions about whether or not you should continue taking your regular medications.

9. Be Aware of Drug Interactions

As a patient, you cannot rely solely on your doctor and pharmacist to stay aware of the possible interactions among your medications. If you assume that your doctor is checking every medication you are taking for interactions with your kidney and liver function, or for specific recommended use for elderly patients, you may be mistaken. Pharmacists are also drug experts, and they are usually your last line of defense against medication-induced illnesses. But their role does not eliminate your need to know about the major interactions among your specific medications, especially if you use multiple pharmacies. Using a single pharmacy that has a complete record of your medications is one way a pharmacist can determine if you have been prescribed drugs that may cause harmful interactions with your other medications. Wanting to shop around for the best prices among different pharmacies is understandable, but a trip to the hospital because of negative drug interactions will cancel any financial savings you may have gained.

10. Understand That Over-the-Counter Medicines, Herbals, and Alcohol Are All Drugs

Another danger is over-the-counter (OTC) medicines. These commonly used substances have the ability to interact with your prescription drugs. Many of these OTC products contain lower doses of prescription-only formulations and come with the same usage concerns. Herbal products, even completely natural formulations, should be considered drugs. For example, ginseng and ginko biloba can decrease the metabolism of warfarin and thus increase the risk of bleeding. Alcohol, too, is a drug; therefore, you must seriously consider how it can interact with other medications in ways that are detrimental to your health.

11. If Your Health Changes after You Add a New Drug, Think Drug-Induced Disease

If you develop a new symptom after beginning a new medication or adjusting the dosage of an existing one, the change in your drug regimen may be causing your problem. Any new symptom(s) should not be ignored. Contact your physician to determine whether the drug may be causing the new symptoms. Be especially concerned if the problems arose within a short time after the new drug was added and nothing else changed. Always ask your pharmacist about possible side effects from any new medications, and be sure to monitor yourself for any changes.

12. Know That Most Adverse Drug Reactions Are Due to Dosage Issues

Seventy-five percent of adverse drug reactions are due to patients receiving medications in amounts that are on the higher end of the dosage spectrum. Ask your doctor if the dose you are prescribed is appropriate for your age, kidney function, and liver function, as all of these factors should be considered when determining your dose. Believe it or not, many physicians rely on standard manufacturer recommendations when determining a starting dose for patients. Double-check with your doctor and pharmacist to make sure the dose is appropriate for you.

13. Insist on Medication Reconciliation

What if your doctor writes information on your new prescriptions in one section of a hospital chart while a nurse records similar information in a different area of the chart? Or suppose you go home from the hospital with conflicting information about your new and existing prescriptions? These kinds of communication gaps among health professionals can sometimes result in patients receiving a damaging mix of medications. To remedy this situation, the Joint Commission recommends that health professionals put medication reconciliation procedures into practice. The term "medication reconciliation" refers to a specific, formal process of creating a complete, accurate, and current list of all medications a patient is taking and comparing that list to the patient's medical record or medication orders—all to make sure the patient is getting correct dosages regardless of where they are within the health-care system. Reconciling differences between the lists of medications should take place every time patients move from one health-care setting to another.

You can play an important role in the reconciliation process by keeping an up-to-date list of all of the medications, OTC drugs, herbals, or nutritional supplements you take, including dosages, times of usage, and method of delivery. The section in this chapter entitled "What Are You Taking and Why Are You Taking It?" will give you tips on setting up this list. You not only need to create the list, you must also make sure that health professionals refer to it and check for any possible drug interactions that could affect you negatively. Therefore, whenever your drug regimen is altered in any way, be sure to ask your doctor, pharmacist, nurse, and other caregivers to double-check your list against their data and insist that they engage in medication reconciliation to protect your health.

What Are You Taking and Why Are You Taking It?

One action that can help support you in following the "16 Rules of Safe Medication Use" is simply this: Keep an up-to-date list of all the medications you take. This list should include information such as the name of the drug, dosage, frequency, and appearance—and you should update it any time your prescriptions are changed. This list can be produced in whatever format works easiest for you—using pen and paper, a computer spreadsheet, or an online application (app) in your mobile phone or other electronic device. The main thing is that you and your family members should have access to the list and present it whenever you interact with the health-care system. As pointed out in Rule #13, it is important to have your list ready when asking clinicians and other health professionals to undertake the "medication-reconciliation" process—that is, to formally compare your list of medications to others they are using to check for the possibility of any adverse drug reactions.

The chart opposite will give you an idea of what your medication list can look like. This sample form, "My Medicine Record," is produced by the Food and Drug Administration (FDA) and can be found at http://www.fda.gov/downloads/AboutFDA/ReportsManualsForms/Forms/UCM095018.pdf. A blank copy of this document is located on page 269, and you should feel free to use it for making your list.

---

14. Don't Stop Taking a Medication Without Talking to Your Doctor

Your doctor placed you on your medications for an important reason, and taking these drugs can help prevent disease complications. It can be harmful to your body if you decide to suddenly discontinue taking a drug, so it is important to talk to your doctor if you are considering stopping any or all of your medications, even if you

MY MEDICINE RECORD

Name (Last, First, Middle Initial): _____   Birth Date (mm/dd/yyyy): _____

	What I'm Using (Rx—Brand and generic name; OTC—Name and active ingredients)	What It Looks Like (color, shape, size, markings, etc.)	How Much	How to Use/When to Use	Start/Stop Dates	Why I'm Using/Notes	Who Told Me to Use/How to Contact
Ex 1	Furosemide	20 mg pill; small, white, round	40 mg; use two 20 mg pills	Take orally, 2 times a day, at 8:00 AM and 8:00 PM	1-15-11	Lowers blood pressure; check blood pressure once a week; blood test on 4-15-11	Dr. X (800) 555-1212
Ex 2	Phenytoin (generic for Dilantin)	100 mg, pink capsule	100 mg, 1 cap	Take orally, once at bedtime	1-21-11	For seizures	Dr. J. (800) 555-8000
3							

These are my medicines as of (Enter date as mm/dd/yyyy): _____

[Source: www.fda.gov/Drugs/ResourcesForYou/ucm079489.htm / [888] INFO-FDA / www.fda.gov/usemedicinesafely / FORM FDA 3664 [3/11]]

Examples added by author.

A blank copy of this form is included on page 269 and may also be downloaded from the entry for this book at www.hunterhouse.com.

are experiencing bad side effects or cannot afford the medications. Your doctor can advise you whether or not it is safe for you to discontinue the drug(s) in question.

15. Remember That Elderly Individuals Should Be on Lower Doses

Rule #15 is a companion to Rule #4, which states that elderly individuals are different from younger people. Their bodies do not function in the same way; thus, the ability of the body to remove a drug through the kidneys or liver may be impaired in older adults. Generally speaking, elderly patients need to be on lower doses to compensate for this decrease in functioning and for various other reasons. Ingesting high doses of medications can make elderly people more vulnerable to increased side effects because of their age. If you are an elderly patient, make sure you are on the correct dose, even if your kidney and liver lab values are within "normal" ranges.

16. Ads Don't Warn of Incidence of Adverse Events—Don't Believe Them

I believe it is the manufacturers' duty to provide the public with information about the incidence of adverse reactions associated with their medications, either through their advertising or through specific warnings on products. The advertisements, however, are usually intended to give people hope for relief of their symptoms without identifying the number of complications that can result from taking the drugs. How many times have you seen people laughing or smiling in a commercial and you can't figure out what the advertised drug is supposed to treat? Commercials often instruct you to contact your doctor if you experience certain symptoms or suggest that this medication may not be an option for you, but this is all said so quickly that you are often left without a realistic view about your risk of experiencing an adverse reaction. Because drug company advertisements usually do not provide enough information to help you seriously consider whether you should take certain medications or not, and not enough warnings are made public, you need to take action to protect yourself.

Protect Yourself: Record and Report

Now that you've read about the 16 rules for using medications safely, I want to underscore why it is so important for you to follow these rules—and also to report any problems you experience when taking drugs. Physicians only report 1 to 10 percent of adverse drug reactions to MedWatch, so the FDA is pushing for consumers to directly report reactions online.[2] To report any adverse events resulting from human health-care products, go to http://www.fda.gov/medwatch/report/consumer/consumer.htm.

Keep in mind that health-care products include OTC and prescription drugs; medical devices (such as contact lenses and glucose tests); blood, human cell, and tissue products (except for vaccines); nutritional products (dietary supplements, infant formulas, and nutritional supplements); and cosmetics.[3] If you have experienced an adverse event, be sure to keep notes to document what happened and report it to the FDA. By doing so, the FDA can become more aware of various drugs' effects and make adjustments to how they are prescribed and monitored, or even withdraw them from the market. Reporting is the most important thing you can do to protect yourself and others. Consumers will not be aware of the potential harm drugs might cause if no one reports their adverse events.

When the media alert the public about highly dangerous road intersections, people usually slow down and drive more cautiously. Warning signs may be erected. The following thirty cases that you will read about in the rest of this book should be thought of as the top thirty dangerous "intersections" where good drugs can have dangerous, unintended effects This book functions in the same manner as those warning signs on a roadway, and it also educates you regarding where you can conduct your own research and learn about any cautionary information related to your medications.

CHAPTER 2

Are Your Meds Causing Problems in the Lungs or Heart?

Most people do not realize that medications can damage the lungs and heart. Some can cause the lungs to swell and damage lung tissue. Other medications have been reported to cause heart failure, irregular heartbeats, and high blood pressure.

███████ **CONDITION** ███████

Medication-Induced Lung Disease

The following case shows us that some medications can cause lung disease. Lung disease is any condition in which lung function is impaired.

THE PATIENT

Wendy is a sixty-five-year-old woman battling heart failure, atrial fibrillation (an irregular heartbeat), high blood pressure, high cholesterol, and gout. She exists on a "diet" of coffee and cigarettes. She has one thing going for her—not a day goes by that she doesn't get out of her home to take a walk with her husband. She is not afraid to pull on that spandex and go for a jaunt around the neighborhood.

THE SYMPTOMS

Over the past few years, Wendy has become short of breath on her walks and has started coughing up a lovely shade of yellow mucus, leaving her husband "not so breathless." These symptoms have been getting worse over time. Wendy has not returned to the doctor or gone in for her lab tests in a while. In the past, she went to see her doctor when these symptoms arose and was prescribed a round of antibiotics to treat her for infection. The antibiotics provided only minimal improvement, and the symptoms kept getting worse. Her difficulty in breathing and her coughing spells have continued to worsen, even when she is inactive. Wendy has also noticed that she is tired all the time and has difficulty going on simple walks. So whose fault is it? What could be causing these symptoms?

THE SUSPECTS

The likely suspects are the following drugs.

1. Nicotine (Cigarettes)

Approximately 20.6 percent of the U.S. population smoked cigarettes in 2005.[1] Nicotine has recreational use in the form of cigarettes, cigars, or chewing tobacco, and it is included in products designed for quitting smoking, such as patches, gum, or lozenges. Nicotine can cause taste changes, upset stomach, high blood pressure, faster heartbeat, bronchitis, emphysema, chronic obstructive pulmonary disease (COPD), and various kinds of cancers.

Tobacco smoke is noxious to the lungs and causes chronic inflammation, damaging the tissues and narrowing the airways. Eventually, the airflow in and out of the lungs becomes restricted. Tobacco smoke can also paralyze the *cilia*, or little hairlike structures, in the airways. The cilia normally move in a wavelike motion to help clear out mucus and other foreign material from airways. If the cilia are paralyzed by cigarette smoke, the lungs can't clear out foreign material, possibly causing the person to be more susceptible to infection.[2]

2. Amiodarone (Trade Names: Cordarone, Pacerone)

Amiodarone is used to treat abnormal heart rhythms (arrhythmias). It can also cause such side effects as low blood pressure (hypotension; 16 percent), slow heartbeat (3–5 percent), tremors, dizziness, fatigue, poor coordination, nausea/vomiting (10–33 percent), abnormal liver tests (4–9 percent), pulmonary fibrosis (4–9 percent), visual disturbances (2–9 percent), and halo vision (up to 5 percent). (The percentages correspond to the number of patients out of 100 that experience a particular side effect.) According to the black box warning on the packaging, amiodarone has the potential to cause serious lung damage at an estimated frequency of 2 to 7 percent and as high as 10 to 17 percent. (Required by the FDA as its strongest warning, a black box label indicates that the medication has the potential to cause a serious or even life-threatening adverse effect.)[3]

Toxicity may be present as hypersensitivity pneumonitis and/or pulmonary fibrosis, which is a gradual buildup of scar tissue in the lungs from chronic irritation and damage. This condition is fatal 10 percent of the time. Amiodarone may also cause severe liver toxicity (damage to the liver) and may also have proarrhythymic effects (causing irregular heartbeat). Dosage must be started in the hospital to make sure the medication is not going to cause another type of irregular heartbeat.

3. Metoprolol (Trade Names: Lopressor, Toprol XL)

Metoprolol treats high blood pressure, heart failure, and heart attacks, and it sometimes helps prevent chest pain (angina). It blocks beta-receptors in the heart and kidneys, slowing the heart rate. Metoprolol can cause a slow heartbeat (2–16 percent), dizziness (10 percent), sleepiness (10 percent), rash/itching (5 percent), shortness of breath (3 percent), decreased exercise tolerance, and cold fingers and toes. Metoprolol also includes a black box warning. The drug should *not* be stopped abruptly. The dosage of Metoprolol needs to be reduced gradually over one to two weeks to avoid exacerbation (worsening) of symptoms, such as increased chest pain and possible heart attack (MI, or myocardial infarction).[4]

LET'S RECAP

Patient: Wendy, age 65

1. Nicotine (cigarettes): 1½–2 packs per day for years

2. Amiodarone (Cordarone, Pacerone) for Irregular heartbeat: 400 mg daily
3. Metoprolol (Lopressor, Toprol XL) for high blood pressure: 50 mg 2 times daily

Lab-test results: Not applicable

X-ray findings: Lung mass on chest CAT scan and X ray

 ### SUMMARY REPORT

An initial evaluation of the situation suggests that Wendy's medical condition is not directly causing the symptoms and that the following information must be considered:

- From the clues, we can determine that metoprolol is not the likely cause of Wendy's symptoms, because she is on a low dose. Metoprolol only affects the bronchioles and airways at high doses.

- The doctor ordered a computerized axial tomography (CAT) scan of the chest. CAT scans are cross-sectional images of the internal organs that provide more detail than conventional X rays. To picture a CAT scan, think about slicing through the chest at an angle parallel to the ground and looking down on that image. For example, if a CAT scan were taken of the feet, it would look like footprints. The doctor decided to get a CAT scan of Wendy's chest. The lungs are usually dark masses, and any infiltrates (bacteria, fibrosis, or anything else abnormal) show up as light areas within the lungs. The damage is usually described as having a glassy appearance, which is what Wendy's doctor saw when he reviewed the results of her CAT scan.

- He also ordered a chest X ray to look at Wendy's lungs. Again, the doctor saw white, cloudy infiltrates within the dark areas.

- Long-term use of nicotine from tobacco products can cause emphysema and chronic bronchitis. In emphysema, the walls of the small terminal air sacs in the lungs are destroyed, causing the air spaces to enlarge. An X ray of lungs with emphysema would reveal these enlarged air spaces, which were not seen. Chronic bronchitis is inflammation of the *bronchioles*, or the two main airways that branch into each lung. An X ray of lungs with chronic bronchitis would show inflammation of the bronchioles, which was not present.[5] Therefore, we can rule out nicotine as the culprit.

SOLVE THE MYSTERY

From the clues, we just ruled out nicotine and Wendy's cigarette smoking as the cause. We also ruled out metoprolol. What's left?

The Culprit: Amiodarone

One of the most severe adverse effects of amiodarone is lung disease. It can cause the lungs to become inflamed, a condition called pneumonitis, and lead to scarring of the lung tissue, which is called pulmonary fibrosis. When lung tissue scars, it hardens and cannot do its normal job of transferring oxygen to the blood. Hence, the person has trouble breathing. X rays of Wendy's chest revealed areas of consolidation (firm masses within the lung) that positively correlate with amiodarone-induced lung disease.

The diagnosis of amiodarone toxicity relies on excluding other possible causes. The clue that a disease is not causing the lung symptoms allows the physician to consider that amiodarone is the culprit.[6]

Amiodarone toxicity can present as interstitial pneumonitis, bronchiolitis, acute respiratory distress syndrome, or pulmonary fibrosis, with interstitial pneumonitis being the most common. The presence of any of these conditions basically means the lungs have been damaged and scarring has occurred. The alveoli and bronchioles now are damaged and will never function the same way. The damage is permanent, but if it had been found earlier, Wendy's lung damage could have been stopped sooner. Now it is too late, as the damage cannot be reversed.

The Accomplice: Nicotine (Cigarette Smoke)

Studies have shown conflicting evidence as to whether preexisting lung damage, which could be caused by chronic nicotine use, puts the person at a higher risk of developing amiodarone-induced lung disease. It is considered a risk factor.[7] Regardless, smoking is bad for your lungs.

 THE SOLUTION

Wendy was admitted to the hospital to be monitored while she stopped taking amiodarone. After a few days, she was able to go home, but her lung function will never be perfect again. If she has problems with her arrhythmia (irregular heartbeat), her doctor will start her on a new drug, such as digoxin, which should not cause the problems she has experienced with amiodarone. Because amiodarone stays in the body for a long time, her physician wants her to go without any similar drug for a while. The doctor also gave her some corticosteroids, a medication to reduce inflammation, to take short term. Her doctor is hopeful that these drugs will help open her lungs and give her some relief.

WHAT ARE YOUR CHANCES?

Adverse reactions causing pulmonary lung disease occur in about 5 percent of patients receiving a drug, and 0.03 percent of hospital deaths are due to drug-related lung disease.[8] In 1972 only 19 drugs had the potential to cause lung disease, but today that number has grown to more than 350 different medications. Amiodarone is the most common drug related to cardiovascular pulmonary toxicities.[9] More than two million prescriptions were written for amiodarone in 2006.[10] Studies have reported that incidence rates of amiodarone-induced lung toxicity can be as high as 10 to 17 percent with doses greater than 400 mg daily, according to the black box warning.[11] From this data, we can reason that at least fifteen thousand people could have developed amiodarone-induced lung toxicity in the year 2006. If you are on chronic amiodarone therapy, you should be aware of this very real adverse reaction. (2,000,000 Rxs/12 Rxs per year for 1 patient = 166,667 patients × 10 percent incidence = 16,667 cases of lung toxicity.) However, a search of MedWatch's database shows only approximately 101 reported pulmonary events during 2007. With two million prescriptions written annually, one would expect more than 16,000 adverse reactions, yet with only 101 cases of pulmonary issues being reported to the FDA, this problem is not being recognized.[12] Lung toxicity is most commonly seen in men older than age forty. Risk increases with age, preexisting lung disease, and dose/duration of amiodarone.[13]

HELPFUL ADVICE

If you are taking amiodarone, this potential complication should be taken seriously. As you can see, lung disease associated with this medication is not a rare occurrence. A patient should be aware of this possibility and know the signs and symptoms to reduce its impact on their quality of life. This case could have been prevented by Wendy taking a different drug such as digoxin. This reaction is a known effect of amiodarone, and avoidance is the only prevention tool. If problems are detected and stopped early, damage may not be significant, but if amiodarone use is continued, the damage it does to the lungs may not be reversible.

The threat of amiodarone-induced lung toxicity peaks in the first year of treatment, regardless of the dose.[14] Some case reports show the toxicity developing months after discontinuing the drug.[15] To stop this toxicity from developing, I recommend getting pulmonary function tests, including DLco (diffusion capacity of lung for carbon monoxide) and a chest X ray, before starting amiodarone and every three to six months thereafter.[16] Patients who are at risk of developing lung toxicities include people who have been on the medication for a long amount of time and are on doses higher than 400 mg a day, but adverse effects may also be seen at doses as low as 200 mg a day.[17] If you are on a dose higher than 400 mg, be on the lookout. As a patient, you should self-monitor for such symptoms as shortness of breath, nonproductive cough (a cough that does not produce any mucus or sputum), chest pain, weight loss, fever, and fatigue. The most common of these are cough and increased shortness of breath.[18] If any of these symptoms occur, contact your doctor. Early detection is the key, because the drug's effects may be minimized if caught early.[19] Amiodarone is not considered first-line therapy, and other options such as digoxin may be a better choice. This medication is reserved for life-threatening arrhythmias and for those who can't benefit from other antiarrhythmics.[20] Talk with your doctor to determine whether another antiarrhythmic can be used in place of amiodarone.

 VIOLATION OF RULE #6: *Know Your Lab-Test Schedule*

Try not to exceed a maximum daily dose of amiodarone of 400 mg, because quantities above this dose have been associated with an increased rate of adverse events. Amiodarone patients should have their lung function (spirometry, diffusing capacity, chest radiograph, CT scan, serum kL-6/MUC1 concentrations[21]) and thyroid function checked before they begin therapy and then checked again every three to six months thereafter.

CONDITION

Medication-Induced Pneumonia

The following case shows us that some medications are capable of causing pneumonia. Pneumonia is an inflammation of the lungs usually caused by infection.

 THE PATIENT

Judy is a stubborn eighty-one-year-old woman who loves tradition. She thinks she has normal problems for her age. She has some trouble with her blood pressure and experiences a little heartburn, and sometimes her hands and her feet cramp up. She does her best to keep these symptoms under control with her medicines. Judy is not able to get out much anymore, but she likes to keep everything she can on a regular schedule. She has had the same daily routine for the last fifty years, and, like her mother always taught her to do, she ingests at least a glass of mineral oil every evening before bed to keep her digestive system moving.

THE SYMPTOMS

Lately, Judy has been slowly becoming increasingly short of breath. She also has a nonproductive cough. She has been experiencing weight loss, having lost about fourteen pounds in a few months, most likely due to some malabsorption. She is starting to get worried about the changes in her health, so she has gone to her doctor.

THE SUSPECTS

The likely suspects are the following drugs.

1. Lorazepam (Trade Name: Ativan)

Lorazepam is usually used for anxiety but also may be used for insomnia, sedation, nausea, alcohol withdrawal, and seizure activity. It can cause dizziness, sedation (≥ 10 percent), vertigo or general unsteadiness, depression (≥ 10 percent), confusion, changes in appetite, and weight gain/loss. Lorazepam is in the class of medications known as the *benzodiazepines*, which may be addictive. It is a controlled substance.[22]

2. Lisinopril (Trade Names: Prinivil, Zestril)

Lisinopril treats high blood pressure and heart failure. It also improves survival after a heart attack and diabetes. It is known to cause low blood pressure (1–10 percent), dizziness (5–12 percent), headache (4–6 percent), dry cough (4–9 percent), and diarrhea (3–4 percent). A known side effect of this drug is its ability to cause a dry, hacking cough. The drug includes a black box warning about taking it during pregnancy, because angiotensin-converting enzyme

(ACE) inhibitors can cause injury and death to a developing fetus when used in the second and third trimesters. Discontinue ACE inhibitors as soon as pregnancy is detected. Lisinopril ranked at number thirteen on the list of most commonly dispensed prescriptions in the U.S. market in 2006, with 25,548,000 scripts.[23]

3. Mineral Oil (Trade Names: Kondremul, Liqui-Doss)

Mineral oil relieves constipation. It may also cause malabsorption of fat-soluble vitamins (some vitamins won't be absorbed from the diet when you take mineral oil regularly) and loose stools. This drug may be swallowed or taken as an enema. The usual dose is 1 to 3 tablespoons before bed, but Judy ingests 1 or 2 cups, probably averaging well over three times the normal dose. Mineral oil can be aspirated (breathed into the lungs when it is supposed to go down the food pipe) and cause pneumonia or lung inflammation.

LET'S RECAP

Patient: Judy, age 81
1. Lorazepam (Ativan) for anxiety: 1 mg 3 times a day as needed
2. Lisinopril (Zestril or Prinivil) for high blood pressure: 10 mg daily
3. Mineral oil as a laxative: 1 or 2 cups in the evening
Lab-test results: Not applicable
X-ray findings: Chest X ray showed something in lung

SUMMARY REPORT

An initial evaluation of the situation suggests that Judy's health problems are not directly causing the symptoms and that the following information must be considered:

- A CAT scan was ordered, and it revealed an abnormality called "crazy-paving," which looks like a pattern of gray circles within the lungs. A normal picture of the lungs would show this area being completely dark.

- The cough usually associated with lisinopril is a dry cough caused by nerve reactions. Once again, Judy has been taking her lisinopril for quite some time and has never had any problems with it before. A cough from lisinopril would most likely present within the first few months of treatment.

- Judy has been taking the lorazepam for a few years now but has never had any weight gain/loss issues with it before.

SOLVE THE MYSTERY

It is doubtful that lisinopril is the culprit, because Judy has been taking this drug for quite some time. If she were to have a reaction to this medication, it would not likely have a rapid onset and probably would have shown up a long time ago. Judy has also been taking the lorazepam for a while and has not had any previous problems while taking it...so what is the culprit?

The Culprit: Mineral Oil

Judy has been taking mineral oil for so long and in such high amounts that she couldn't help but have a little bit accidentally go down the wrong pipe and into her lungs. Aspiration doesn't necessarily lead to problems for most people, because the body can usually get rid of the foreign substance by coughing it up; however, this does not occur with mineral oil, because it soothes the throat as it goes down, thereby stopping the normal cough reflex (which happens when we accidentally breathe something in, such as water). The body does not know what to do with the oil, so it gets stuck and can cause pneumonia.[24] This pneumonia is known as chemical pneumonitis, which is an inflammation of the lungs due to an irritant.[25] It is also known as lipoid pneumonia, which is caused by an aspiration of lipids (such as fats or oils).[26]

THE SOLUTION

Judy was treated by stopping her consumption of mineral oil. Over time, her body will slowly get rid of it, but she may develop some scarring in the lungs. Her doctor had tried prescribing antibiotics before finding the mineral oil in her lungs, but that did not help her condition. If her condition had been more severe, the doctor could have put her on oxygen until she recovered. A procedure for severe cases basically washes out the lungs.

WHAT ARE YOUR CHANCES?

Pneumonia caused by mineral oil is extremely rare. Most cases go undetected, because they do not produce any major problems. Data from an autopsy series suggested an incidence of 1 to 2.5 percent. In a study of 389 mainly neurologically ill patients at risk of this type of pneumonia, the incidence was 14.6 percent.[27] No recent studies have been conducted that give a true incidence that would relate to today's use; additionally, different age groups have different factors that might increase their chances of developing pneumonia. Some factors that increase your chances of developing pneumonia include your ability to swallow, malfunctions with your digestive tract and stomach, the amount of mineral oil that you use, and the number of days you have been using it. These factors make you more likely to develop a problem, especially if you are very young or elderly.[28]

HELPFUL ADVICE

Mineral oil is not used as commonly anymore, because companies are always developing and marketing newer products to treat digestive concerns. If you are taking mineral oil, this complication should not worry you too much. However, it is wise to talk with your doctor or pharmacist about some safer options for constipation to determine which one is the best option for you. These products include stimulant laxatives (Senokot, Dulcolax), stool softeners (docusate [Colace]), and bulk-forming laxatives (Metamucil, Citrucel). After extensive research, no negative incidence could be found, so it is reasonable to assume mineral oil is safe to consume when caution is exercised to reduce possible lung ingestion. In the future, Judy should remember Rule #10 and recognize that over-the-counter (OTC) products are still drugs and have possible adverse effects.

Patients who are at risk of lipoid pneumonia should not use mineral oil. These patients include children and elderly patients with neurological disease, patients who have a hard time swallowing, and patients with gastroparesis and gastrointestinal reflux disease. Patients should not use mineral oil prior to lying down or sleeping.[29] Even if they are not at risk, they should not use mineral oil for more than a week.[30]

Other oil-based products, such as liquid paraffin for or oil-based nose sprays, may also cause this problem when being used to coat the mouth or nose or when swallowed. Avoid any oil-based products to prevent pneumonia from occurring.

 ### VIOLATION OF RULE #10: Understand That Over-the-Counter Medications, Herbals, and Alcohol Are All Drugs

Mineral oil is an OTC medication that most patients believe cannot hurt them, but even the most innocuous medication should be used with caution. In this case, mineral-oil ingestion can lead to pneumonia, and it can also cause decreased absorption of vitamins and other medications, such as warfarin or oral contraceptives. Mineral oil should not be used in elderly patients or patients with disabilities due to the risk of aspiration (breathing into the lungs) and pneumonia.

 ### VIOLATION OF RULE #15: Remember That Elderly Individuals Should Be on Lower Doses

If you have frequent constipation, try nonmedication methods first. Drink two to three quarts of fluid a day, exercise as tolerated, and increase the amounts of fruits and vegetables in your diet, especially fiber.[31] If these options do not work, you may want to try Metamucil, Citrucel, Docusate, or Miralax, which are safer and can be used long term. Talk with your doctor or pharmacist to see which option is best for you. It is important that elderly people take the lowest dose, which would be 15 ml of mineral oil at bedtime.[32]

■■■■■■■■ CONDITION ■■■■■■■■

Medication-Induced Respiratory Insufficiency (Breathing Problems)

The following case shows us that some medications can cause respiratory insufficiency. Respiratory insufficiency is the condition in which there is insufficient breathing to maintain proper bodily functions.

THE PATIENT

Bernie is a seventy-one-year-old retired truck driver. Driving was his life for thirty-five years, and now it seems that his body is breaking down, just like his old rig. He always said some people weren't cut out for life on the road, but now it looks as though Bernie isn't cut out for life on the couch.

THE SYMPTOMS

Bernie had back surgery last week and is still laid up in the hospital. The surgeon has weaned him off his morphine pump and switched him to tablets in preparation for his trip home. Bernie doesn't mind, because he had not been using the pump very often. His first dose of oral morphine put him to sleep for five hours in the middle of the day. That wasn't a problem, because he usually has trouble sleeping when he isn't in his rig. After two more doses, though, he has begun to experience difficulty breathing. Bernie has started feeling very agitated and breathless, so he is insisting on seeing the doctor immediately.

THE SUSPECTS

The likely suspects are the following drugs.

1. Morphine Extended-Release (Trade Name: MS Contin)

Morphine relieves severe pain but can cause nausea and vomiting (7–70 percent), vision changes (<5 percent), constipation (>10 percent), skin rashes/itching (up to 80 percent), respiratory depression

(4–7 percent), and drowsiness (>10 percent). It is a controlled substance (meaning that strict regulations control its use to ensure it is not being abused), and it has a high abuse potential. Patients should not abruptly stop treatment, because withdrawal symptoms may occur. A black box warning states that extended-release tablets are not intended to be crushed. Breaking these tablets eliminates the timed-release mechanism and delivers the entire dose immediately, which could lead to an acute overdose.[33]

2. Benazepril (Trade Name: Lotensin)

Benazepril decreases blood pressure. It can also cause such side effects as dry cough (1.2–10 percent), hypotension (low blood pressure; <1 percent), decreased kidney function (2 percent), hyperkalemia (1 percent), dizziness (3.4 percent), and fatigue (2.4 percent). This medication includes a black box warning. Use in the second or third trimester of pregnancy is absolutely contraindicated, as benazepril can cause fetal birth defects. This medication has also been found to cause an allergic-type reaction in the face, lips, tongue, and throat, known as angioedema, that may be life-threatening.[34]

3. Hydrocodone and Acetaminophen (Trade Names: Lortab, Vicodin, Norco)

Hydrocodone and acetaminophen work to relieve moderate to severe pain. They can cause nausea and vomiting, vision changes, constipation, low blood pressure, skin rashes, respiratory depression, drowsiness, and memory impairment. Hydrocodone is a controlled substance and has a high abuse potential. Patients should not stop treatment abruptly, as withdrawal symptoms may occur. Patients should take other acetaminophen-containing products with caution while on this combination. The maximum recommended dose is 4,000 mg daily. At higher doses, acetaminophen can cause serious and sometimes irreversible damage to the liver. It is important to ask your doctor or pharmacist about any medications that may contain acetaminophen to be sure you are not taking too much.[35]

LET'S RECAP

Patient: Bernie, age 71

1. Morphine ER (MS Contin) for pain from recent surgery: 60 mg 2 times daily
2. Benazepril (Lotensin) for high blood pressure: 20 mg daily
3. Hydrocodone/acetaminophen for chronic lower back pain as needed (Lortab, Vicodin, Norco): 10/500 mg* every 8 hours

Lab-test results:

O₂ saturation: 78 percent (normally 90–100 percent; less than 90 percent is low)

Blood pressure: 78/41 (normally 120/80 or below)

SCr (serum creatinine): 3 mg/dL (normally 0.6–1.4 mg/dL)

BUN (blood urea nitrogen): 18 mg/dL (normally 7–18 mg/dL)

X-ray findings/other tests:

Respiratory rate: 4 breaths per minute (normally about 14–18 breaths per minute)

---

* 10/500 is the appropriate way to express the dosage for a combination drug. It reflects that the drug contains 10 mg of hydrocodone and 500 mg of acetaminophen.

SUMMARY REPORT

An initial evaluation of the situation suggests that Bernie's back problems are not directly causing the symptoms and that the following information must be considered:

- Bernie is on two pain medications that may affect breathing.
- Bernie is experiencing low blood pressure.
- His oxygen saturation is 78 percent, but it should be over 94 percent.
- His respiratory rate is only four breaths per minute (the normal rate is about twenty per minute).

SOLVE THE MYSTERY

Bernie is not doing very well. He was ready to go home, but now it appears that he will have to stay until the problem can be solved. Looking at the evidence, we see three possible suspects. Benazepril seems a likely culprit, because it causes a dry cough. However, it is not the guilty party this time, because no cough was ever present. Then we have Bernie's longtime use of hydrocodone and acetaminophen. Although these medications do not appear to have been the ones that pulled the trigger, let's keep an eye on them anyway. Finally, we have morphine, which was just recently added. It appears he may have left too many clues at the scene of the crime.

The Culprits: Morphine

It looks like this is another case of excess. In higher doses, opioids, such as morphine, can cause respiratory depression. Although the exact reason is not known, these drugs are thought to basically shut down the sensors that detect a buildup of carbon dioxide in the blood. Carbon dioxide is the waste gas that the body produces when it breaks down food for energy. As with a car and its exhaust system, the human body has to rid itself of carbon dioxide. When this waste increases in the body, the brain usually tells the lungs to breathe deeper and faster to get rid of the excess. When drugs or injury shut down this mechanism, a person can die. This is why immediate medical attention is always needed in the case of a possible opioid overdose.[36]

The Accomplices: Hydrocodone and Acetaminophen

Although hydrocodone and acetaminophen have been there all along, they are not innocent in this matter. The acetaminophen can claim no wrongdoing though, as all the bad reactions here resulted from the hydrocodone. Hydrocodone is also an opioid, and together with morphine it can have additive adverse effects, such as Bernie's respiratory depression. To a trained eye, it was evident from the start that this combination of drugs was to blame. Bernie was not using his morphine pump much but was given a large dose of long-acting morphine anyway. These two drugs, prescribed in excessive amounts, can cause the anxiety and breathlessness Bernie experienced due to the lack of drive from the brain to breathe. These symptoms create an impending sense of doom for a patient, a very unpleasant experience. Hydrocodone can be used with morphine, but dosing and timing must be carefully monitored.

THE SOLUTION

In this situation, Bernie should be carefully removed from these drugs. A slow, gradual decline from these two drug doses will reduce the risk of withdrawal symptoms due to Bernie's long-term therapy on hydrocodone, which may have made him physically dependent on it. After this withdrawal, we are hopeful that Bernie will not need any further pain medication. He had surgery to correct his back problem. From the lack of pain he experienced immediately after the surgery, we are hopeful his medicated days are over.

WHAT ARE YOUR CHANCES?

The number of people experiencing respiratory depression during opioid therapy is only 0.5 to 2 percent. However, with about 155 million prescriptions dispensed for hydrocodone, morphine, and oxycodone products in 2007, those percentages translate into 65,000 to 260,000 patients who could be affected. Respiratory depression is a very real reaction, and patients need to be aware of it. Those most likely to have this problem are elderly and seriously ill patients in hospital intensive care units, because of complex drug regimens.[37] (155,000,000 Rxs/12 Rxs per year for 1 patient = 12,916,667 patients × 0.5–2 percent incidence = ~64,583–258,333 cases of respiratory depression.) However, as is noted throughout this book, cases of respiratory depression with opiates are not being reported. A search of MedWatch's database revealed only twenty-five reports of shortness of breath, respiratory depression, and respiratory arrest due to morphine sulfate. These reports amount to far less than the expected number of cases occurring on a daily basis in the United States. When looking at the hydrocodone/acetaminophen (Lortab) data available on MedWatch, no apparent respiratory depression reports were available from 2007.[38]

HELPFUL ADVICE

The majority of these cases occur in overdose victims and in patients taking high doses of opioids along with other medications that can cause respiratory depression. The average patient on chronic opioid therapy should not worry about this complication under typical circumstances. Any other problems with opioids are much more common and should be dealt with cautiously. In the future, it would help if Rules #2, #4, and #15 were followed instead of being broken as they were in this case. Even though Bernie did not really break any rules, a doctor should have taken his age and previous usage of opioids into account when choosing the dosage level for the morphine tablets.

If you must take a pain medication, such as morphine or hydrocodone, on a regular basis, be wary of any changes in your health. These drugs are highly effective at treating pain but can also cause much toxicity. A change in the way your body eliminates these drugs could cause an unwanted adverse reaction. I recommend having your doctor monitor your GFR rate while on any opioid therapy. (Calculated by your doctor, GFR, or glomerular filtration rate, is a good indicator of how well your kidneys are working.) A patient experiencing kidney problems should not use codeine, meperidine, or propoxyphene.[39]

Opioids must be taken with caution and recognition of the serious consequences of abusing these drugs. "Unintentional drug overdose is the second leading cause of accidental death in the United States, just behind automobile crashes. According to the Centers for Disease Control and Prevention (CDC), between 1999 and 2004 the number of overdose deaths in the United States rose 77 percent, to almost 20,000. The CDC attributes the 62.5 percent rise in drug overdose deaths between 1999 and 2004 to a higher use of prescription painkillers and increasing numbers of overdoses of cocaine and prescription sedatives."[40] A person is also at higher risk of overdosing if they use multiple medications and/or mix prescription drugs, illegal drugs, and alcohol. Try to use just one medication to manage your pain and at the lowest dosage to prevent the occurrence of overdose.

VIOLATION OF RULE #2: Know Your Kidney Lab Values

The patient's SCr (serum creatinine) is 3, which is elevated and which makes it difficult for his body to get rid of the morphine and hydrocodone.

VIOLATION OF RULE #4: Be Aware That Elderly Patients Are Different from Younger People

The patient taking the morphine and Loritab is elderly—seventy-one years old. Elderly patients should have the status of their respiratory systems monitored closely when on high doses of opiates. Patients like Bernie, who was in a hospital setting, are at a disadvantage when it comes to knowing their prescribed doses and frequencies, but this is no excuse. As a patient in the hospital, you have the right to receive information about your treatment, and you can always ask to see your chart and lab values.

VIOLATION OF RULE #15: Remember That Elderly Individuals Should Be on Lower Doses

As explained in Chapter 1, lab values are important when it comes to adjusting the doses of medications, especially in elderly patients whose kidney or liver functioning may be declining. Always double-check with your doctor to make sure the dose isn't too high. The dose of the oral morphine you should be given when you go home should be *half* the dose you were given while on the morphine pump.[41] The dose of your pain medication should be lowered to an effective dose if you are being switched from intravenous morphine to oral morphine, especially if you are an elderly patient and are prone to its side effects. Besides elderly patients, other individuals who should proceed with caution while on morphine are patients with hypothyroidism, adrenocortical insufficiency, impaired kidneys, increased prostate, obstructive bowel disorder, shock, or myasthenia gravis, and those who are also taking monoamine oxidase inhibitors (for example, Marplan and Nardil).[42]

As for hydrocodone and acetaminophen, elderly patients should be on 2.5 or 5 mg of the hydrocodone component every four to six hours.[43] If you take your pain medications and they cause cold, clammy skin, confusion, convulsions, drowsiness, low blood pressure, restlessness, pinpoint pupils, or trouble breathing, contact your doctor immediately—these are side effects of an overdose. Do not crush or chew time-released tablets, and do not combine other depressants, such as alcohol, pain relievers, sleep medications, tricyclic antidepressants (for example, amitriptyline), or phenothiazines (such as chlorpromazine or thioridazine), because this can cause overdosage or an exaggerated central nervous system depression to occur.[44]

■■■■■■■ **CONDITION** ■■■■■■■

Medication-Induced Cough

*While most people are familiar with the soothing effects
of cough syrup, the following case shows us that some
medications can cause a chronic cough.*

THE PATIENT

Evan drives a school bus for the local school district. He is an active forty-one-year-old. He likes to bowl in a league on Tuesday nights. He also coaches his twin sons' basketball team. About a month or so ago, he went to his family doctor for an annual physical. The doctor checked his blood pressure and performed the usual exams. He also wanted to check Evan's cholesterol, so he ordered a lipid profile on his blood tests. Sure enough, it was determined that Evan was suffering from high blood pressure and high cholesterol. This was true even though he has an active lifestyle. The doctor wrote two new prescriptions (fosinopril and simvastatin) for Evan and wanted to see him again in three months for a follow-up appointment.

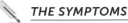

THE SYMPTOMS

Evan starts experiencing an annoying cough. Cold season does not usually affect Evan, and he doesn't smoke. The cough seems different from any cough he has had before with a cold. No mucus is clogging his head or lungs: It is a dry cough that keeps him awake at night and is very bothersome. So he decides to see his doctor after six months to see what is causing the horrible cough.

THE SUSPECTS

The likely suspects are the following drugs.

1. Simvastatin (Trade Name: Zocor)

Simvastatin decreases cholesterol by decreasing the amount of cholesterol the body can make. Constipation (2 percent) and headache (1 percent) are the most common side effects. Some people experience muscle pains that can indicate serious problems with muscle breakdown. Other medicines for cholesterol may increase the chance of these muscle pains. This medicine is also combined with ezetimibe in a combination tablet (Vytorin).[45]

2. Fosinopril (Trade Name: Monopril)

Fosinopril is used for the treatment of high blood pressure, congestive heart failure, and left ventricular dysfunction after a heart attack. Dizziness (2–12 percent) is the main side effect seen with fosinopril, which should decrease as patients become used to the medicine. Other possible side effects include low blood pressure when the patient stands up (1–2 percent), headache (3 percent), fatigue (1–2 percent), high potassium (2–3 percent), diarrhea/nausea/vomiting (1–2 percent), and cough (2–10 percent).

Fosinopril belongs to a class of medications known as ACE inhibitors. The class of ACE inhibitors also includes many other commonly prescribed drugs, such as lisinopril (Zestril, Prinivil), captopril (Capoten), ramipril (Altace), enalapril (Vasotec), quinapril (Accupril), and moexipril (Univasc), to name a few. This means the drug works to inhibit an angiotensin-converting enzyme (ACE).

This enzyme causes another substance to be made that can increase blood pressure in a couple of ways. So someone taking an ACE inhibitor is preventing the increase in blood pressure caused by a substance known as angiotensin II. All ACE inhibitors work the same way, so they all have the same adverse reaction profile. A black box warning on ACE inhibitors says they should not be taken during pregnancy, as they can cause injury and death to a developing fetus when used in the second and third trimesters. Discontinue ACE inhibitors as soon as pregnancy is detected.[46]

3. Ibuprofen (Trade Names: Advil, Motrin)

Ibuprofen reduces pain and inflammation or swelling, but it can also cause abdominal pain (1–3 percent), heartburn (3–9 percent), ringing in the ears (3–9 percent), and edema or fluid retention (1–3 percent). Ibuprofen belongs to a class of drugs called nonsteroidal anti-inflammatory drugs (NSAIDs) and may increase the risk for heart attack or stroke. A black box warning states that ibuprofen may increase the risk of cardiovascular events and increase risk for GI bleeding or ulceration.[47]

 LET'S RECAP

Patient: Evan, age 41
1. Simvastatin (Zocor) for high cholesterol: 20 mg at bedtime
2. Fosinopril (Monopril) for high blood pressure: 20 mg daily
3. Ibuprofen (Advil or Motrin) for inflamed/painful knee: 400 mg
   3 times a day
Lab-test results: All normal
X-ray findings: Chest X ray was normal

 SUMMARY REPORT

An initial evaluation suggests that the disease is not causing the symptoms and that the following information must be considered:

- The simvastatin and fosinopril were the new drugs prescribed for Evan.

- Evan has been on ibuprofen since he was thirty and has not experienced any problems.

- Evan has no signs of infection, such as a fever or increased mucus production.
- Simvastatin has not been reported to cause cough.

SOLVE THE MYSTERY

The clues pretty much spell out what is going on. The only medication left is fosinopril.

The Culprit: Fosinopril

Evan's description of his cough fits his symptoms. ACE inhibitor–induced cough is usually described as a dry, nonproductive, hacky cough that is often worse when a patient lies down at night.[48] The cough generally appears early after starting ACE inhibitor therapy but could present several months later. ACE inhibitor–induced cough can be often misdiagnosed, and other causes of cough need to be excluded.[49] Some other causes of cough may be infection related, smoking induced, or related to another lung disease. The severity of the cough is dependent on the patient and varies greatly. In some instances, the cough is not bothersome enough for the patient to discontinue the medication.

THE SOLUTION

If the cough is severe enough, the most effective way to alleviate it is to discontine the ACE inhibitor. Once this is discontinued, it may take a couple of days or up to a month before the cough disappears. The physician will generally not select another drug from the ACE inhibitor class and will utilize another class of antihypertensive agents. This reaction is what is known as a "class effect." This means that if a patient has a reaction on one ACE inhibitor, they will most likely have the same reaction to another ACE inhibitor.

WHAT ARE YOUR CHANCES?

ACE inhibitors as a class ranked number nine of the top ten therapeutic classes by sales in 2004, with $4.4 million in sales recorded.[50]

In 2006 25.5 million prescriptions were dispensed in the United States for lisinopril (ACE inhibitor) alone.[51] As of January 24, 2008, the U.S. population was approximately 303 million people,[52] which means that approximately 8 percent of Americans were on lisinopril, just one of the drugs in this class. The incidence of drug-induced cough while on an ACE inhibitor depends on which one you are taking. Captopril has a rate of about 2 percent, while ramipril can be as high as 12 percent.[53] The incidence of cough due to an ACE inhibitor overall has been reported to be 3 to 20 percent,[54] so let's take the average, which is 11.5 percent. If 25.5 million people are on lisinopril and 11.5 percent have the possibility of experiencing the cough, 2.9 million patients could experience this side effect. Also, as previously mentioned, this cough does not always cause the patient to stop taking the medication, but it is reported that cough leads to about 5 percent of patients stopping the medication,[55] which is equal to about 145,000 people discontinuing lisinopril due to drug-induced cough. That is 1 in 2,089 people, which is just a little better than your chances of fatally slipping in a bath or shower.[56] (2,656,000 fosinopril Rxs in 2007/12 Rxs per year for 1 patient = 221,333 patients × 3–20 percent = 6,640–44,267 cases of cough/ year.) According to the FDA's MedWatch system, in 2007 only four cases of cough were attributed to fosinopril use. Most likely, many cases of ACE inhibitor cough go unreported, because it is a common adverse drug reaction.[57]

HELPFUL ADVICE

This reaction is extremely common among patients taking ACE inhibitors, and it seems to be more common in women than men.[58] The elderly (people more than sixty years old) and Chinese, Japanese, Indians, and African Americans are more susceptible to this reaction.[59] Because the drug is one of the leading classes of medications, this problem is an extremely large issue for the general public. If you are started on an ACE inhibitor and develop a cough, chances are high that you have been afflicted with this issue.

Abiding by the "16 Rules of Safe Medication Use" would not have helped Evan in this case. ACE inhibitor–induced cough is an adverse reaction that has no predisposing risk factors, lab tests, or monitoring parameters to prevent it from happening. This is a common, well-known adverse effect from ACE inhibitors, and the only prevention is avoiding the medicine; however, given ACE inhibitors' usefulness in reducing blood pressure along with cardiovascular and renal problems, avoiding ACE inhibitors in prescribing practice is unwise.

If you experience a cough soon after starting an ACE inhibitor, think drug reaction. This cough usually begins several months after initiating the drug but may show up as early as the first dose or as late as one year. The cough may diminish within three days and disappear within ten days of stopping the offending drug.[60] OTC cough medications will not usually alleviate this cough and may lead to additional drug interactions. It is important to make an appointment with your doctor if you are bothered by this dry cough, but do not suddenly stop taking your medication. Your doctor may be able to prescribe another medication, such as an angiotensin receptor blocker (ARB). These drugs include losartan, irbesartan, telmisartan, valsartan, and olmesartan and are not usually associated with drug-induced cough.

 VIOLATION OF RULE. None

Evan was a victim of an adverse reaction that neither he nor his doctor or pharmacist could have prevented. However, Evan did suffer from this persistent cough for six months before notifying his doctor. Always realize that medications could be the cause of medical problems. ACE inhibitors offer amazing benefits for cardiovascular and renal disease and should not be avoided just because they can cause a cough. If a dry cough does arise, consult your doctor or pharmacist, who may suggest a medication that works in nearly the same fashion, such as an ARB (angiotensin receptor blocker). The ARBs have not been associated with the same incidence of cough as ACE inhibitors, and they work on the same pathways in your body. They are, however, still brand-name medications, which makes them a much more expensive option. ACE inhibitors should remain a first-line treatment for high blood pressure and prevention of cardiovascular disease.

▬▬▬ CONDITION ▬▬▬

Medication-Induced Arrhythmia

The following case shows us that some medications can cause a change in your heart's rhythm. An arrhythmia is a change in the rhythm of the heart.

THE PATIENT

Thelma is awesome. There is really no other way to describe her. She is seventy-eight years old and has a great social life. She still lives at home with her husband, and she works part-time volunteering at a nursing home. She and her husband go dancing on Mondays and play bingo on Wednesdays, and every Thursday she plays cards with her bridge club and he has his poker night. Thelma's mind is still sharp as a tack, too, but her heart isn't as strong as the rest of her. She had a heart attack about fifteen years ago. She takes medications for her heart, including metoprolol and hydrochlorothiazide. She tolerates her meds pretty well; they don't give her much trouble. But she has had some problems with her sinuses this spring that she thought were just allergies but turned out to be a sinus infection. She went to see her doctor, who prescribed Levofloxacin 500 mg daily for ten days.

THE SYMPTOMS

About four days after seeing the doctor, Thelma starts having arrhythmic heart episodes. They happen especially after she gets up from sitting or from lying down, and it feels like her heart is beating almost out of her chest. She also gets very dizzy, and she thinks she may have once blacked out for a moment. She and her husband were scared, because they were afraid she was having another heart attack. After an episode where she almost falls on the floor, Thelma and her husband hustle over to the ER. She waits a couple of hours, and when she gets back to an exam room she isn't feeling very well again. The ER doctors hook her up to a cardiac monitor and verify that she isn't having another heart attack, but she is experiencing a type of heart arrhythmia called *torsades de pointes*.

THE SUSPECTS

The likely suspects are the following drugs.

1. Metoprolol (Trade Names: Lopressor, Toprol XL)

Metoprolol is used for the treatment of high blood pressure, heart failure, heart attacks, and sometimes the prevention of chest pain. Some side effects include slow heartbeat (2–16 percent), dizziness (10 percent), sleepiness (10 percent), rash/itching (5 percent), shortness of breath (3 percent), decreased exercise tolerance, and cold fingers and toes. Metoprolol works by blocking beta-receptors in the heart, thus decreasing the heart rate. A black box warning states that users should avoid stopping metoprolol abruptly. Use of this drug needs to be tapered off gradually over the course of one to two weeks to avoid exacerbation (worsening) of symptoms, such as worsening of chest pain.[61]

2. Hydrochlorothiazide (Trade Name: Microzide)

Hydrochlorothiazide is a diuretic (thiazide) and works by removing excess fluid for hypertension and edema control. It can cause hypotension and dizziness (1–10 percent), electrolyte imbalances (hypokalemia; 1–10 percent), photosensitivity/sunburn (<1 percent), and allergic reactions (sulfonamide; <1 percent). A warning should pop into the patient's head concerning this medication, because it can cause electrolyte imbalances (hypokalemia), allergic reactions, photosensitivity, and gout attacks, and it may be ineffective in patients with a creatinine clearance of <30 mL/min.[62]

3. Levofloxacin (Trade Name: Levaquin)

Levofloxacin is a broad spectrum antibiotic, so it can fight off many different types of bacteria. It is typically used for respiratory infections, urinary tract infections, and skin infections and can cause headache (6 percent), insomnia (4 percent), and dizziness (3 percent). Levofloxacin can cause central nervous system (CNS) stimulation (anxiety, confusion, depression, and hallucinations), tendon rupture, *C. difficile*–associated diarrhea, and QT interval prolongation (cardiac arrhythmias). Elderly patients are more susceptible to adverse events.[63]

LET'S RECAP

Patient: Thelma, age 78
1. Metoprolol succinate (Toprol XL) for hypertension: 50 mg daily
2. Hydrochlorothiazide (Microzide) for hypertension: 25 mg daily
3. Levofloxacin (Levaquin) for sinus infections: 500 mg daily for 10 days

Lab-test results:
    Heart rate: 110 bpm (normally 60–100 bpm)
    Blood pressure: 108/76 mmHg (normally 120/80 mmHg)
    Potassium (K): 3.5 mEq/L (normally 3.5–5.2 mEq/L)

SUMMARY REPORT

An initial evaluation of the situation suggests that Thelma's heart condition is not directly causing the symptoms and that the following information must be considered:

- Thelma is seventy-eight years old. Medically she's considered elderly, even if she wouldn't agree with the term.

- Her potassium is on the low end of normal. A normal range is 3.5 to 5 mEq/L, and we like to see readings around 4 mEq/L.

- From looking at the suspect list, we know that:
    – Elderly patients are more prone to side effects, such as cardiac arrhythmias, from levofloxacin.[64]
    – Metoprolol shouldn't cause her any problems with a fast heartbeat. It should only slow her heart down.

– Hydrochlorothiazide causes hypokalemia, and hypokalemia can cause irregular heartbeats, but she has been stable on this dose for a long time. What is the new medication?

SOLVE THE MYSTERY

Although the condition is rare, Thelma is predisposed to arrhythmias from her heart attack a few years ago. She has been sick, and she has not been eating and drinking enough, so her potassium is somewhat low. Her lower potassium combined with an arrhythmia-producing drug equals torsades de pointes.[65]

The Culprit: Levofloxacin-Induced Torsades de Pointes (Arrhythmia)

When the heart doesn't beat correctly, it is called an arrhythmia. To understand the type of arrhythmia called torsades de pointes, you first have to understand how the heart beats. You must consider two separate aspects: the mechanical part and the electrical part.[66]

The Mechanical Part

The actual flow of the heartbeat is pretty complicated, and if it doesn't happen just right, many problems can occur. See if you can follow the blood flow in the heartbeat in Figure 2.1. The medium gray areas signify blood without oxygen, and the light gray areas signify freshly oxygenated blood [67]

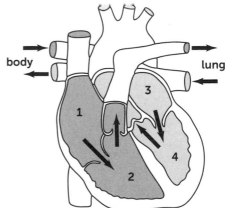

1. Right atrium: Blood coming from the body (blood that needs oxygen) comes here first.

2. Right ventricle: The right ventricle pumps blood to the lungs where it can get oxygen.

3. Left atrium: Freshly oxygenated blood comes into the left atrium from the lungs.

Figure 2.1. The flow of blood in a heartbeat

4. Left ventricle: This chamber pumps oxygenated blood out to the body.

The Electrical Part

When the heart beats, everything contracts and relaxes in a specific sequence. Electrical impulses control that sequence. Now it is kind of strange to think about, but these electrical impulses happen all by themselves. That is, the brain doesn't tell the heart to beat.

There are many different types of arrhythmias, including one type called ventricular tachycardia, in which the ventricles (#2 and #4 in Figure 2.1) beat faster than the atria (#1 and #3). This situation is bad for many reasons, mostly because the atria can't empty all the way and the ventricles can't fill up all the way. Torsades de pointes is a specific type of ventricular tachycardia.

Torsades de pointes happens because of a prolongation of the QT interval. The QT interval describes a specific contract/relax relationship in the heart, and if the interval lasts longer than normal, torsades de pointes can result. A person can be born with a long QT interval, or medications or electrolyte disorders can cause it. Levofloxacin is one of the medications known to cause QT prolongation, and hypokalemia is an electrolyte imbalance known to do the same thing.

The Accomplice: Low Potassium (Hypokalemia)

Thelma says she hasn't been eating well or staying hydrated as well as she should. However, she is still taking her hydrochlorothiazide. Hydrochlorothiazide makes users excrete potassium, and because she isn't taking in much potassium, her potassium levels have been a little low. A potassium level that is too low puts patients at a higher risk of developing an arrhythmia.[68]

THE SOLUTION

Thelma is very lucky, because in some patients, one incident of torsades de pointes can cause instant death. Thelma's heart is able to reset itself and beat normally again, but every time she has an episode, she's in danger of dying. Her heart resets itself again when she is in the ER, but not before the doctors identify the problem.[69]

Because her episodes are drug-induced, she will not have to take medications to prevent torsades de pointes in the future, but she will have to avoid the medications that could cause it. She is taken off the levofloxacin immediately and receives counseling on the importance of proper nutrition and hydration during illness. She also is given a list of medications that have been linked with torsades de pointes and is warned to tell her present and future medical doctors that this reaction occurred.

WHAT ARE YOUR CHANCES?

Levofloxacin is in a drug class called quinolones. Other quinolones include Cipro (ciprofloxacin), Avelox (moxifloxacin), Floxin (ofloxacin), and Tequin (gatifloxacin).

Between January 1, 1996, and May 2, 2001, 25 cases of quinolone-induced torsades de pointes were identified and reported in a medical journal entitled *Pharmacotherapy.*[70]

ciprofloxacin = 2 cases

ofloxacin = 2 cases

levofloxacin = 13 cases

gatifloxacin = 8 cases

moxifloxacin = 0 cases

However, in 2007 there were 15 cases of torsades de pointes, arrhythmia, and prolonged QT interval attributed to levofloxacin that were reported to the FDA and posted on the MedWatch site.[71]

HELPFUL ADVICE

As mentioned earlier, this arrhythmia is a rare occurrence. However, to decrease your chances, ask your physician and pharmacist if any medications you are on affect older patients differently from younger patients. If Thelma had followed Rule #4, she may have avoided this problem.[72]

If you notice a change in your heartbeat when you are taking levofloxacin, document the changes and try to describe them. If you think your heart isn't beating in rhythm, is beating too fast, or feels as though it is "beating out of your chest," or if you're experiencing fainting episodes or symptoms like those Thelma experienced, let your doctor know.[73]

Older women are more at risk than other adults for quinolone-induced torsades de pointes. In general, the quinolones may not be the best choice for the elderly, because that population is more prone to developing adverse events, such as headache, insomnia, dizziness, CNS stimulation, tendon rupture, and *C. difficile* diarrhea. If you or a loved one is over sixty-five years old and is prescribed a quinolone, double-check with your doctor that the benefits outweigh the risks. Risk factors that can predispose you to torsades de pointes include heart complications, having low potassium and magnesium levels, being older, being female, having a low heart rate, being on more than one drug known to cause torsades, possibly being genetically predisposed, or having a previous history of torsades.[74]

Several other medications should be used cautiously because of their risk of causing torsades de pointes, such as several antiarrhythmics (for example, quinidine, disopyramide, procainamide, sotalol, dofetilide, ibutilide, bepridil, and amiodarone), psychotropic drugs (for instance, chlorpromazine, thioridazine, mesoridazine, pimozide, and haloperidol), antibiotics (such as erythromycin and clarithromycin), and miscellaneous drugs (such as methadone, pentamidine, levomethadyl, halofantrine, droperidol, chloroquine, and cisapride). If you are experiencing any changes in heart rhythm, you can always go to the following website to determine whether your drug may be causing this effect: http://www.azcert.org/medical-pros/drug-lists/list-01.cfm.

The website lists drugs that carry a risk, drugs that have a possible risk, and drugs with a conditional risk associated with torsades de pointes. You can then alert your doctor of this association if it is likely that torsades is occurring.

You can take a few preventative actions, such as having your QTc interval monitored and having your serum potassium and magnesium levels checked and maintained above 4 mEq/L and 2 mEq/L, respectively. (The QT interval is the measure of time between the onset of ventricular depolarization and completion of ventricular repolarization. The QTc interval is the QT interval corrected for the heart rate.) Adjust the doses of these medications based on your renal and kidney function, and watch for drug interactions with the medications you are on.[75]

VIOLATION OF RULE #4: Be Aware That Elderly Patients Are Different from Younger People

Thelma is lucky. She had her husband there to recognize the serious problems she was having with her heart. Like many other patients, Thelma had a reaction that is more common in older patients. As people age, their bodies become more sensitive to some medications, such as quinolone antibiotics. If you're an older patient, you should always ask your physician and pharmacist whether your prescribed medications cause any serious side effects that show up more frequently in older adults.

VIOLATION OF RULE #11: If Your Health Changes after You Add a New Drug, Think Drug-Induced Disease

Thelma should have also realized that her fainting and heart problems could have been due to the new medication she was taking. Any new problems that arise shortly after adding a new medication should immediately cause you to consider the possibility that the disease or condition is drug induced.

Are Your Meds Causing Kidney, Calcium, Liver, Pancreas, or Diabetic Complications?

Medications can cause problems in areas that many people would not suspect. Hospital admissions occur daily for people that suffer medication-induced kidney, liver, and pancreas problems, as well as medication-induced diabetes.

▰▰▰ CONDITION ▰▰▰

Medication-Induced Renal (Kidney) Failure

The following case shows us that there are a number of medications that can cause renal failure. Renal failure is a condition in which the kidneys do not work well or cease to function at all on their own.

THE PATIENT

George is a fifty-year-old man living vicariously through his son's basketball career. He was never much of an athlete himself in his younger days, and now he is disabled due to multiple injuries requiring surgeries. He has been diagnosed with high blood pressure, insomnia, and peripheral vascular disease.

THE SYMPTOMS

It is the middle of basketball season, and George hates to miss a play, let alone a whole game. He has to get up and run to the restroom very frequently, and consequently he's missing some great plays by his very own shooting guard. He recently had the flu and was vomiting and had a bout of diarrhea for four days. He is now feeling nearly back up to speed, but he has noticed that he is not producing much urine when he tries to use the restroom. Not only is it an annoyance; urinating has also become very painful for him. What is going on with George's apparent bladder problem?

THE SUSPECTS

The likely suspects are the following drugs.

1. Etodolac (Trade Name: Lodine)

Etodolac is used for the management of pain and arthritis. Side effects include dyspepsia (upset stomach; 10 percent), nausea and vomiting, diarrhea, flatulence, abdominal cramps, weakness (3–9 percent), rash, ringing in the ears, water retention, and anemia (1–3 percent). It may also cause stomach ulcers after long-term use.[1]

Etodolac belongs to a class of drugs called nonsteroidal anti-inflammatory drugs (NSAIDs). Up to 5 percent of people taking these drugs are admitted to the hospital for renal (kidney) toxicity each year.[2] Etodolac has a less than 1 percent incidence of renal failure. Its black box warning says it can increase the risk of cardiovascular events and risk for GI (gastrointestinal) bleeding or ulceration.[3]

2. Amlodipine (Trade Name: Norvasc)

Amlodipine is used to treat high blood pressure, chronic chest pain (angina), and vasospastic (Prinzmetal's) angina and to prevent hospitalization due to chest pain with coronary artery disease. It belongs to the class of medications known as calcium channel blockers (CCBs). These medications help make the heart's workload easier by reducing the resistance the heart has to pump against in the arteries. It ranked fourth on the list of most prescribed drugs in 2006, with more than forty million prescriptions written.[4]

The most commonly seen adverse reaction that occurs with amlodipine is peripheral edema (swelling in the arms/legs/ankles, and so forth; 2–15 percent). Other reactions include headache (7 percent, but this figure is similar to that from the placebo, which is 8 percent), flushing (1–3 percent), rapid heartbeat (1–4 percent), itching/rash (1–2 percent), nausea (3 percent), and pulmonary edema (15 percent, from PRAISE trial) in patients with congestive heart failure. (More than 1,000 patients with severe chronic heart failure participated in the PRAISE trial to determine the effects of amlodipine [1996, *New England Journal of Medicine*].)

3. Trazodone (Trade Name: Desyrel)

Trazodone is used as an antidepressant and sleep aid. Antidepressants potentially increase suicidal thoughts. Trazodone can cause prominent drowsiness and sedation, so doctors prescribe it at bedtime for insomnia. It can cause dizziness (>10 percent), headache (>10 percent), sedation (>10 percent), blurred vision (>10 percent), hypotension (low blood pressure; 1–10 percent), and priapism (prolonged erection; <1 percent), just to name a few conditions. A black box warning states that trazodone may increase suicidal thoughts in children or adolescents. It ranked seventy-first on the list of most commonly dispensed prescriptions in the U.S. market in 2006.[5]

LET'S RECAP

Patient: George, age 50
1. Etodolac (Lodine) for inflammation: 300 mg daily
2. Amlodipine (Norvasc) for insomnia: 50 mg at bedtime
3. Trazodone (Desyrel) for insomnia: 50 mg at bedtime
Lab-test results:
    SCr(serum creatinine): 3.2 mg/dL (normally 0.6–1.4 mg/dL)
X-ray findings: Not applicable

SUMMARY REPORT

An initial evaluation of the situation suggests that George's various health problems are not directly causing the symptoms and that the following information must be considered:

- George recently had his yearly prostate exam, and everything was reported to be normal. He has no prostate enlargement.

- George's kidney function was tested a while back, and he was found to have a serum creatinine of 1.0 mg/dL, which is normal. When he comes in this time, after his bout with the flu, it measures 3.2 mg/dL. Creatinine is a protein created from muscle breakdown and is normally released into the blood at a constant level due to normal cell replacement. Increased levels indicate that his kidneys are not eliminating it at a normal rate.

- The problem could be due to a combination of his medication with his recent flu episode.

- Amlodipine has rarely been associated with nocturia, or increased urination at night...could this be the problem?

- George recently started taking more etodolac than prescribed due to his muscle aches from the flu.

- If it isn't his prostate, which we might have initially thought was the culprit considering his symptoms (frequent urination)...what is the culprit? Etodolac or amlodipine?

 SOLVE THE MYSTERY!

Even though it is a common cause of these types of symptoms in older men, we know that George's prostate isn't causing his symptoms, because he recently had his checkup. George is taking an NSAID, which might be responsible for kidney failure. He also recently had an episode of the flu that could have had an effect. Use the previous clues to solve the mystery yourself. Be careful...it is a little tricky!

 The Culprit: The Combination of Etodolac and Dehydration

As mentioned previously, etodolac is classified as an NSAID. NSAIDs can reduce blood flow to the kidneys, thereby reducing their ability to filter the blood. When this is combined with dehydration, as seen with the flu, kidney damage becomes a real possibility. George started taking more etodolac for his muscle aches, which has only worsened the problem. NSAIDs reduce the production of molecules called prostaglandins in the body. Reducing these prostaglandins is what leads to both the good and bad effects of NSAIDs.[6] In this case, the reduction of prostaglandins has had a bad effect on the kidneys. Normally, prostaglandins are released to allow more blood flow to the kidneys. Etodolac stops these prostaglandins from being produced. Combining more than the recommended dose with George's dehydration has only further reduced the amount of blood his kidneys are getting. Therefore, an additive reduction in renal perfusion (or blood flow to the kidney) is seen. It produces a condition known as renal insufficiency. Basically, it means George's kidneys aren't getting enough blood flow to properly filter the waste from his blood.[7]

THE SOLUTION

George begins receiving another drug for his pain. The etodolac is switched to acetaminophen (aka Tylenol), which is the only non-NSAID over-the-counter (OTC) pain reliever. Drug-induced acute renal failure can often be prevented. Health-care providers should avoid combinations of drugs that are associated with inducing renal failure. It may also be necessary to start medications such as these with low doses and continue to monitor renal function.

WHAT ARE YOUR CHANCES?

It has been reported that drugs are responsible for 20 percent of hospitalizations for acute renal failure. The incidence of acute renal failure varies, but the number of people admitted to the hospital is about 5 percent.[8] This means approximately seventy-six thousand people are admitted with drug-induced acute renal failure a year. (38,000,000 hospital admissions × 1 percent = 380,000 patients × 20 percent incidence = 76,000 cases of renal toxicity.) NSAIDs are the most widely used drugs in the United States.[9] Up to fifty million people in the United States use NSAIDs at any time, and about 1 to 3 percent of users may experience renal toxicity.[10] If 3 percent are experiencing toxicities, that comes out to 1.5 million Americans who may possibly be diagnosed with some sort of renal failure and are being treated for a drug reaction that mostly can be prevented. In a study, 18 percent of patients who received ibuprofen developed acute renal failure, and another study revealed 13 percent acute renal failure in an elderly population using NSAIDs.[11] Patients taking etodolac (Lodine) report a less than 1 percent chance of incurring renal failure. In the last four quarters of 2007, only three cases of acute renal failure associated with etodolac were reported to Med-Watch.[12] This data is only for etodolac, but it still grossly underestimates the total number of cases from NSAIDs seen in the United States that year.

HELPFUL ADVICE

This drug-induced disease is not a rare occurrence and should be treated seriously. NSAIDs can increase the incidence of acute renal failure by four times, requiring hospitalization during the first month of therapy.[13] The major problem here is patients taking NSAIDs in unsafe amounts. When the patient is dehydrated and then starts taking a drug that may cause kidney problems, the risk of developing renal failure greatly increases. Knowing George's kidney lab values and monitoring parameters and him taking his medications as directed would have eliminated the problem before it resulted in a trip to the ER. Trazodone is eliminated by the kidneys as well, but fortunately George is on the correct dose.[14] Trazodone is on the list of drugs that are preferred in the elderly, and his dosage of 50 mg at bedtime is appropriate.

If you already have problems with your kidneys, be careful when taking OTC medicines, because they may decrease your kidney function. If you are like George, who did not have any prior kidney problems, be careful when taking more than one medicine that may cause kidney problems, and be aware of any increase in symptoms. Also, if you are sick and dehydrated, don't continue taking your medications, because doing so can lead to more damage to your kidneys. Kidney specialists suggest stopping your medications and calling your doctor immediately to determine how best to proceed.

If you are over the age of sixty-five, exercise caution while taking NSAIDs. Your kidney function may already be compromised, and taking this medication can cause further problems. Other risk factors leading to acute renal failure from NSAIDs include being an elderly man, taking a high dose of NSAIDs, having cardiovascular disease, experiencing recent hospitalization for nonrenal disease, and using other drugs that can be harmful to the kidneys.[15] I do not recommend the use of NSAIDs in these patients, so other alternatives should be used, such as acetaminophen.

If you're taking OTC NSAIDs, do not take them for more than ten days because of the risk of damage to your kidneys and gastrointestinal ulcers/bleeding. Don't take NSAIDs if you know you're dehydrated or your lab results for kidney function show damage. Drinking a large glass of water while taking NSAIDs may help flush out the drug but may not help stop declining kidney function. Further damage can occur to your kidneys if you drink caffeine while on NSAIDs, so avoid drinking any caffeinated beverages while on these medications.[16]

Other drugs that may cause renal dysfunction include angiotensin-converting enzyme (ACE) inhibitors, angiotensin receptor blockers (ARBs), cyclosporine, tacrolimus, rifampin, loop diuretics, thiazide diuretics, proton pump inhibitors, phenytoin, lithium, aminoglycosides, amphotericin B, cisplatin, acyclovir, methotrexate, and allopurinol.[17]

If you experience any of the following symptoms of acute renal failure, contact your doctor immediately: swelling of the legs and feet, little or no urine output, pain in the lower back, confusion/anxiety, thirst, rapid heart rate, loss of appetite, drowsiness, headache, nausea and vomiting, and dizziness.[18] If you think you are suffering from renal toxicity, stop taking your drugs, but be sure to seek immediate assistance and consultation from your physician.

VIOLATION OF RULE #2: *Know Your Kidney Lab Values*

Remember that OTC medications, such as naproxen and ibuprofen, are NSAIDs, which means they are drugs, too. Even OTC ibuprofen in low doses can alter kidney function. Illness can change your hydration status and therefore kidney function as well. Always check with your doctor and pharmacist before increasing any medication or starting an OTC medication for an illness. Have your renal function checked, if possible, and make sure your kidney lab values are within the appropriate ranges.

VIOLATION OF RULE #6: *Know Your Lab-Test Schedule*

Had George been vigilant with his lab-test schedule, which includes a test for renal function, he and his doctor would have detected this problem earlier. If you are on an NSAID, you should have your urine output and CHEM-7 (includes SCr [serum creatinine], BUN [blood urea nitrogen], Na [sodium], and K+ [potassium], among others) lab test performed before you start taking the medication and then repeating the lab tests every three months thereafter.

VIOLATION OF RULE #7: *Know Your Medication's Monitoring Parameters*

Avoid NSAIDs if you're a patient with chronic kidney disease with a SCr level >1.7 mg/dL or liver disease, and if you're a member of another high-risk population (elderly, diabetic, heart-failure, or dehydrated patients). If NSAIDs must be used, use them for a short duration (three to five days) or use another agent, such as acetaminophen. NSAIDs should be discontinued if SCr, BUN, or K+ levels increase. Avoid using NSAIDs while on other drugs that may affect the kidneys, including diuretics, ACE inhibitors, and ARBs, especially if you are elderly and have high blood pressure or heart failure.[19]

━━━━━ **CONDITION** ━━━━━

Medication-Induced Hypercalcemia (Excessive Calcium)

The following case shows us that some medications can cause hypercalemia. Hypercalcemia is the presence of abnormally high levels of calcium in the blood.

THE PATIENT

Jim is an upstanding citizen involved in his community, even at the age of seventy. He usually goes to bingo and other community activities at the local senior center. He considers himself fairly healthy for his age, despite the doctor's telling him that he has high cholesterol and high blood pressure. He also has some chronic knee pain, which he attributes to old age. Being the conscientious man that he is, he takes his medicines just as his doctor prescribes them. Just for good measure, he also drinks milk three times a day and takes his multivitamins along with fish oil (omega-3 fatty acids) every day. Several times a day Jim has heartburn, so he always has his Tums Ultra (calcium carbonate–based antacid) around. He guesses that he takes at least five to ten of these a day.

THE SYMPTOMS

Lately Jim has been having problems keeping up, and he finds himself needing to take frequent catnaps. Sometimes, he gets light-headed and dizzy when he stands up. He also is a little worried about the weight he has gained recently. He has not been eating a lot because of nausea. He has tried to keep drinking at least the same amount of water. His heartburn has been feeling better due to his excessive use of calcium carbonate (Tums Ultra), but what is causing all these other problems?

THE SUSPECTS

The likely suspects are the following drugs.

1. Simvastatin (Trade Name: Zocor)

Simvastatin reduces cholesterol by decreasing the amount the body can make. Even though it has positive effects, it doesn't come without negative ones. Constipation (2 percent) and headache (1 percent) are the most common. Some people experience muscle pains (myopathy) that can develop into a serious problem with muscle breakdown. Other medicines for cholesterol may increase the incidence of these muscle pains. This medicine is also available paired with ezetimibe (Zetia) in a combination tablet (Vytorin).[20]

2. Naproxen (Trade Names: Aleve, Naprosyn)

Naproxen reduces mild-to-moderate pain. It may also be used for the management of ankylosing spondylitis (chronic inflammation of the spine), osteoarthritis (most arthritis pain, due to a degeneration of joints), or rheumatoid disorders (rheumatoid arthritis, arthritis due to an immune response in the joints). Naproxen is also used to treat pain caused by gout, tendonitis, bursitis, dysmenorrhea, or fever. This medication belongs to the NSAID class of drugs, which reduce pain and inflammation. Naproxen works by inhibiting cyclo-oxygenase (COX) and prostaglandin synthesis, which are responsible for pain and inflammation.

Naproxen can cause abdominal pain (3–9 percent), constipation (3–9 percent), heartburn (3–9 percent), headache (3–9 percent), edema (3–9 percent), GI ulceration (ulcer in the stomach intestines, or colon) and bleeding (<3 percent), and kidney problems (renal failure or insufficiency; <1 percent). Jim is taking more than the recommended dose. The recommended maximum daily OTC dose is 600 mg naproxen base per day, or about 3 naproxen tablets.[21]

3. Calcium Carbonate (Trade Names: OsCal 500, Rolaids, Tums)

$CaCO_3$ is calcium carbonate. It is commonly used as an antacid in popular OTC heartburn medicines and in calcium supplements for osteoporosis. Some patients take calcium carbonate (Tums,

Rolaids) for calcium supplementation to prevent heartburn. Up to 10 percent of patients can experience constipation, nausea, dry mouth, decreased appetite, hypercalcemia (elevated blood calcium levels), and increased urination frequency. Jim may take up to ten tablets a day until his heartburn is gone.[22]

LET'S RECAP
Patient: Jim, age 50
1. Simvastatin (Zocor) for high cholesterol: 40 mg in the evening
2. Naproxen (Naprosyn or Anaprox) for inflammation: 440 mg 3 times daily
3. Calcium carbonate (many) for heartburn: 1,000 mg with symptoms of heartburn

Lab-test results:
    Ca (calcium): 14.5 mg/dL (normally: 8.5–10.2 mg/dL)
    SCr (serum creatinine): 1.5 mg/dL (normally: 0.6–1.4 mg/dL)
X-ray findings: Not applicable

SUMMARY REPORT

An initial evaluation of the situation suggests that Jim's health issues are not directly causing the symptoms and that the following information must be considered:

- Jim's calcium value is abnormal, at 14.5 mg/dL. We would like this to be between 8.5 and 10 mg/dL.

SOLVE THE MYSTERY

Jim's calcium was reported to be too high. Hmm…I think it is apparent what the culprit is there.

The Culprit: Calcium Carbonate

This is another case of excess. The guilty culprit is too much calcium carbonate for his body to handle. All of Jim's tiredness and nausea are being caused by an excess of calcium in the body, also called hypercalcemia.

Jim probably needs to take the calcium carbonate in the first place for the heartburn caused by damage to his stomach from the naproxen, a common problem from long-term use of NSAIDs (a case explaining a link between NSAIDs and aspirin and damage to the digestive tract is coming up on page 151).

THE SOLUTION

Jim is admitted to the hospital, where he is given medicine to decrease his calcium level. He is also given a different heartburn medicine that is more effective than the antacid. His naproxen is changed to acetaminophen (Tylenol), which is the only over-the-counter (OTC) non-NSAID pain reliever.

WHAT ARE YOUR CHANCES?

Fifty thousand cases of hypercalcemia occur in the United States each year. Most of these cases are patients with cancer. Approximately 20 to 30 percent of cancer patients experience hypercalcemia at some point.[23] After an exhaustive search, no reported incidence of hypercalcemia due to calcium carbonate (Tums) could be located. It is an OTC medication, and therefore finding data on related adverse events, especially rare adverse drug reactions (ADRs), is difficult. However, three cases of hypercalcemia were reported to the FDA's MedWatch system in 2007.[24] Hypercalcemia is a serious complication of therapy with antacids that can lead to cardiac problems if not caught early.

HELPFUL ADVICE

Hypercalcemia (too much calcium in the blood) is a serious complication that can occur with OTC antacid use. Many people use antacids on a daily basis without thinking of any serious complications; however, the average patient should be concerned when taking such medications, as these potential complications can be extremely serious if not treated properly. In the future, Jim should be taught Rules #5, #6, and #10 for safe medication use. The easiest fix is for Jim to be proactive. If Jim had looked at the bottles and followed the directions, he may have avoided hospitalization. As always, OTC products are drugs and should be respected when used.

Always look on the medicine label for a recommended dose and maximum daily dose. In this case, the maximum dose of calcium carbonate (Tums Ultra) is not to exceed more than seven tablets in a day. The high dosage of calcium carbonate is only supposed to be used for approximately two weeks without the supervision of your doctor. This high dosage needs to be monitored to ensure you are not creating any harmful effects. If you find yourself reaching or exceeding this maximum, talk to your health-care provider, because they may be able to suggest a safer alternative for you.

If you experience nausea, vomiting, changes in mental status, abdominal or lower back pain, constipation, exhaustion, depression, muscle/joint pain, headache, or increased urination, contact your doctor. These are nonspecific signs that may indicate hypercalcemia. The elderly may exhibit more of these symptoms at lower increases of calcium compared to younger adults.[25]

If you have constant or frequent heartburn, see your doctor immediately, because it is possible that you have stomach or esophagus damage. In this case, naproxen may have caused stomach ulceration. Remember to avoid NSAIDs because of the risk of this complication. If needed, use the lowest dose possible for the shortest duration. Do not just cover up a problem with another medication. This doesn't solve the underlying problem, and serious damage can occur. Jim was switched to acetaminophen once the problem was uncovered.

Many nonmedication options can help control heartburn. These include avoiding high-fat foods or any foods that cause heartburn, eating smaller meals, not lying down soon after eating, losing weight, avoiding restrictive clothing, and avoiding alcohol. If these don't help, many medication options treat heartburn, and being educated about these different types of meds may help you figure out which option is the best for you.[26]

Antacid medications quickly neutralize the acid in your stomach. Many different forms of antacids are available. One type is Alka Seltzer, a sodium-containing antacid. This option may not be the best choice if you have high blood pressure or if you are on a sodium-restricted diet. Another kind is calcium-containing antacids, such as Tums. They are not a good idea if you are prone to constipation or already experiencing kidney problems, as calcium carbonate may increase the risk of kidney stones. Magnesium-containing antacids can also cause kidney stones if used for a prolonged amount of time. Examples of these include Maalox and Mylanta. If you take too much of this medication, your blood pressure can drop, which can lead to respiratory or cardiac depression (slowed breathing or heart rate). The last type of antacid is one that contains aluminum, such as Rolaids.

Two more types of medications may be prescribed for heartburn: H2 blockers and proton pump inhibitors (PPIs). H2 blockers prevent acid from being produced; some examples include cimetidine (Tagamet) and Zantac. These should generally be avoided if you have kidney and liver impairment. Exercise caution if you are elderly, have lung disease or diabetes, or are immunocompromised because of the risk of developing community-acquired pneumonia.[27] PPIs block the production of acid more effectively and for longer periods of time. These medications include Prilosec and Nexium. Use with caution if you have liver disease.

Now you are a little more knowledgeable about heartburn medications and may be able to avoid an unfortunate situation. If you have any doubt as to which medication is best for you, always talk to your pharmacist or doctor.

 ### VIOLATION OF RULE #5: Take Your Medications as Your Doctor Prescribed

This problem started with George's taking too many calcium carbonate (Tums) tablets. By ingesting this excess, he created a major medical problem for himself. Always take OTC medications as directed by the label, and be sure to follow any warnings that advise you to check with your doctor before starting to take an OTC product. OTC medications are labeled so they may be used as safely as possible.

VIOLATION OF RULE #7: *Know Your Medication's Monitoring Parameters*

Had George known the monitoring parameters for his medications and been vigilant with his lab-test schedule (which includes a test for calcium levels), he and his doctor would have detected this problem earlier. You should have your calcium levels checked before beginning treatment and then again every three months thereafter to make sure you are not getting too much calcium.

 VIOLATION OF RULE #10: *Understand That Over-the-Counter Medicines, Herbals, and Alcohol Are All Drugs*

Remember that OTC medications, such as calcium carbonate (Tums), are drugs, too. Even OTC antacid use can have serious consequences if not used appropriately. Follow all directions, and if you find yourself needing more than the recommended dose, contact your doctor to discuss trying something else. Check with your doctor and pharmacist before increasing any medication or starting an OTC drug for the illness.

■■■■ CONDITION ■■■■

Medication-Induced Liver Dysfunction

The following case shows us that some medications can cause liver dysfunction. Liver dysfunction is when the liver does not work properly.

 THE PATIENT

Shirley is a fifty-five-year-old hiking enthusiast. She plans her weekends around exploring new hiking routes with her husband. In a few weeks she is going on the longest hike of the year through Yellowstone National Park, if her knees are up to it. She suffers from occasional arthritis in her knees due to her lifetime love of hiking, and she controls this pain by taking Tylenol Extra Strength. Most of the time she does not let this little nuisance interfere with what makes her happy. It is beautiful in the fall, and she is excited about preparing for the trip.

THE SYMPTOMS

Recently Shirley went to the hospital because of the pain in her knees and was prescribed a combination product of hydrocodone and acetaminophen. A few days later, Shirley began to feel weak. She hasn't had much of an appetite and has been feeling nauseated. She decides to wait things out and see if she will feel better; maybe she just has the flu. She doesn't want anything to ruin her big trip, and she is praying she will get well in time. The next day, the right upper part of her stomach is hurting, her symptoms aren't going away, and the weirdest part is that her skin is starting to become yellow. This worries her, so she decides she needs to see her doctor immediately because something is just not right.

THE SUSPECTS

The likely suspects are the following drugs.

1. Acetaminophen (Trade Name: Tylenol)

Acetaminophen is used to treat mild to moderate pain, headache, fevers, osteoarthritis, and dysmenorrhea. Side effects include rash, GI bleeding, and kidney and liver dysfunction. Acetaminophen can cause damage to the liver. To prevent these side effects from happening, patients should not use more than 4,000 mg per day or drink alcohol while using acetaminophen. Watch out for products that may contain acetaminophen combined with other ingredients.[28]

2. Hydrocodone and Acetaminophen (Trade Names: Lortab, Vicodin, Norco)

Products that combine both hydrocodone and acetaminophen are used to relieve moderate to severe pain. Some side effects of this medication are nausea and vomiting, vision changes, constipation, low blood pressure, rashes, respiratory depression (slowed breathing), and memory impairment. Hydrocodone is a controlled substance with a high potential for abuse. Patients using this drug should not abruptly stop taking it, as withdrawal symptoms are likely, and patients should avoid taking any extra acetaminophen while on this medication. Again, the maximum dose of acetaminophen is 4,000 mg a day due to the increased risk of liver damage.[29]

LET'S RECAP

Patient: Shirley, age 55
1. Acetaminophen (Tylenol Extra Strength) for arthritis pain: 2 tablets (500 mg) every 4 hours
2. Hydrocodone/acetaminophen (Lortab, Vicodin, Norco) for arthritis pain: 1–2 tablets (5/500 mg*) every 4–6 hours
Lab-test results:
   AST (aspartate aminotransferase): 78 U/L (usually 5–40)
   ALT (alanine transaminase): 1,011 U/L (usually 7–56)
X-ray findings: Jaundice, enlarged liver

* 5/500 is the appropriate way to express the dosage for a combination drug. It reflects that the drug contains 5 mg of hydrocodone and 500 mg of acetaminophen.

SUMMARY REPORT

An initial evaluation of the situation suggests that Shirley's arthritis and knee pain are not directly causing the symptoms and that the following information must be considered:

- Shirley's liver lab values are elevated, showing liver damage.
- The doctor notices she has jaundice, which is also another sign of liver damage.
- Shirley is on two medications that may cause liver damage.

SOLVE THE MYSTERY

Shirley is admitted to the hospital due to liver damage. What could have caused this to happen? She is on two medications that have the potential to cause this damage. Shirley is already on acetaminophen and then starts on hydrocodone/acetaminophen when the problem happens. Can you solve this one?

The Culprits: Acetaminophen and Hydrocodone/Acetaminophen

Taking just acetaminophen alone can increase the likelihood of having liver toxicities, but adding another medication that also contains acetaminophen greatly increases the risk of this happening. Had Shirley known that she is only supposed to take 4,000 mg of acetaminophen a day and that the combination product also contains acetaminophen, she could have been in Yellowstone Park hiking. The overdose occurred because the liver tries to break down acetaminophen to help the body get rid of the medicine. When this process happens, a toxic compound (NAPQI) is made. Usually another compound, glutathione, binds to this toxic compound, and the combination leaves the body. When the levels of glutathione are not high enough, or if someone ingests too much acetaminophen (which produces so much NAPQI that the glutathione cannot bind it all), NAPQI binds to the cells in the liver and kills them.[30]

THE SOLUTION

Shirley is admitted to the hospital. Her doctor notices her yellow skin and enlarged liver, so he decides to run liver lab tests and a drug urine screen. The lab tests come back positive for acetaminophen toxicity as well as elevated numbers in her liver lab values (AST [aspartate aminotransferase] and ALT [alanine transaminase]). He decides to administer a drug called N-acetylcysteine to replenish the glutathione stores, which will help bind NAPQI and reduce liver toxicity. Luckily for Shirley, the damage is not severe enough for her to be considered for a liver transplant.

WHAT ARE YOUR CHANCES?

More than nine hundred drugs, toxins, and herbs have been known to cause liver damage. About 75 percent of rare drug reactions result in liver transplantation and death, and drug-induced hepatotoxicity is the number-one reason why drugs are withdrawn from the market. In the United States, more than two thousand cases of acute liver toxicity occur yearly, with drugs accounting for more than half of them, and approximately 39 percent of drug-related cases are caused by acetaminophen (780 acetaminophen-induced acute liver toxicity cases a year). More than two hundred million Americans take acetaminophen each year, and more than fifty-six thousand emergency department visits and five hundred deaths each year in the United States result from acetaminophen toxicity. In 1998 the American Association of Poison Control Centers received reports of more than one hundred thousand overdoses involving acetaminophen. According to this organization, excessive use of acetaminophen is one of the most common causes of overdose. Acetaminophen toxicities are the number-one cause of acute liver failure and are the second-most-common reason for liver transplantation. Taking just two Extra Strength Tylenol tablets more than four times a day can cause an overdose, and it only takes a few days to cause liver damage. Case reports show that 4 percent of patients who develop liver toxicities eventually suffer from liver failure; up to half of these patients will need a liver transplant or will die. According to the FDA's MedWatch reporting for three quarters of 2007, eighty-six reports of some sort of liver damage and nine liver transplants for patients only taking acetaminophen were recorded. Three cases of liver damage occurred for patients taking acetaminophen/hydrocodone. These results did not include intentional and accidental overdosage, which likely caused the majority of cases. Liver damage may have occurred in these situations.[31]

 HELPFUL ADVICE

Acetaminophen-induced liver damage includes four phases. If these are caught early, patients can prevent severe liver damage and the possibility of requiring a liver transplant.

- **Phase 1** occurs within 24 hours of accidental or intentional overdose. Signs include nausea and vomiting, sweating, and decreased appetite. Patients don't feel well, so they may take more acetaminophen. Some people may not present any symptoms but still have liver damage.

- **Phase 2** occurs between 24 and 72 hours after the overdose. Phase 1 symptoms may wane or resolve altogether. Pain and tenderness can show up in the upper-right part of the abdomen. Liver enlargement and decreased urine output can occur during this phase. Low blood pressure and increased heart rate may occur. Liver lab values (AST [aspartate amino-transferase] and ALT [alanine transaminase]) and others (bilirubin and prothrombin time) can be elevated as well.

- **Phase 3** occurs between 72 and 120 hours after the overdose. Symptoms in Phase 1 may reappear, and more symptoms of liver failure may be seen (jaundice, bleeding, low blood sugar). Kidney failure and an increased heart size may occur in this phase. Cell death can be seen, and 4 percent of patients in this phase can progress to fulminant liver toxicity (severe liver failure). Death is a possibility because of increased water and pressure on the brain and multiorgan failure.

- **Phase 4** occurs between 5 and 14 days after the overdose and can last as long as 21 days. Patients can completely recover or die from liver failure.[32]

Acetaminophen is the most widely used analgesic and anti-pyretic (fever reducer) in the United States and is found in more than two hundred OTC and prescription products as a single en-tity or in combination.[33] Make sure you are not exceeding 4,000 mg a day of acetaminophen, and check to see which products you are taking contain acetaminophen. Some factors can predispose you to acetaminophen-induced liver toxicity such as age, poor diet, liver disease, malnutrition, gastroenteritis (inflammation of the gastro-intestinal tract), chronic alcoholism, alcoholism, and HIV. These factors affect glutathione stores in the body. If you are suffering from any of these disease states, make sure you are monitoring your acet-aminophen intake. Try to limit your doses or avoid acetaminophen altogether. Some medications also stimulate liver enzymes to pro-duce more toxic acetaminophen byproduct (NAPQI). These drugs are isoniazid, rifampin, phenytoin, phenobarbital, barbiturates, and carbamazepine. If you are on any of these medications, again monitor how much acetaminophen you are taking or avoid overuse. Do not drink alcohol while on acetaminophen, because doing so can greatly increase the chances of liver toxicities occurring. If you are on this medication for an extended amount of time, you may want to have your liver enzymes checked periodically (for example, every three months). Acetaminophen-induced liver toxicity is a major problem with grave consequences. It is preventable, so it is imperative that you check every product you are taking to determine whether it contains acetaminophen. Many OTC medications contain this drug, so watch which products you are choosing.[34]

VIOLATION OF RULE #1: Learn from Others—What Is Happening in the ER?

Many people come into emergency departments with acetaminophen toxicity, and many need liver transplants. This condition is easy to prevent. By making yourself aware of the products you are taking and how much you are ingesting in a day, you can easily avoid this serious problem.

VIOLATION OF RULE #3: Know Your Liver Lab Values

One of the major reasons drugs are pulled from the market by the FDA is because they cause liver problems. Individuals need to know their liver lab values and keep a record of them, because if these values are elevated, there is a greater risk of toxicity.

VIOLATION OF RULE #10: Understand That Over-the-Counter Medicines, Herbals, and Alcohol Are All Drugs

Acetaminophen is a popular OTC medication and is also used in many products that combine drugs to treat multiple problems. As you can see from this case, it is easy for someone to accidentally overdose, causing major liver problems. It is important for you to know that this complication exists and to be aware that acetaminophen is included in many OTC cough and cold products. The label will tell you the active ingredients contained in the medication and how much acetaminophen is in each dose. Drinking alcohol while taking any amount of acetaminophen greatly increases the risk of liver toxicity. Even taking "safe" doses of acetaminophen while drinking alcohol can cause damage. If you plan on drinking, take an NSAID, such as ibuprofen, for pain or fever reduction.

VIOLATION OF RULE #16: Ads Don't Warn of Incidence of Adverse Events—Don't Believe Them

Tylenol commercials air frequently, but none states the incidence of any adverse events. One commercial informs the public of the lower risk of stomach irritation compared with aspirin and NSAIDs but does not list any side effects associated with the use of Tylenol. Small print at the bottom of the screen reads, "Do not take Tylenol with any other products containing acetaminophen," but no information regarding the rate of liver toxicities is offered. These commercials are not clearly informing the public of the chances of this toxicity occurring. You now know that this toxicity is a major source of drug-related adverse reactions and have been warned about the risks of developing liver toxicity and how to prevent this situation from happening.

CONDITION

Medication-Induced Pancreatitis

Pancreatitis, a disease in which the pancreas becomes inflamed, can be exacerbated by certain medications, as the following case demonstrates.

THE PATIENT

Ned loves his beer—every day of the week. What used to be six or seven beers a day has turned into two, maybe three, since he turned fifty years old. The old farmer claims that the liquid courage has never let him down, except the time last week when he fell off his tractor and hurt his hip. Despite the injury, Ned appears to be in excellent shape for age seventy-one. He has, however, been diagnosed with hypertension (high blood pressure).

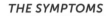

THE SYMPTOMS

Ned is watching NASCAR and eating lunch when he feels a sharp pain in his abdomen. He becomes very nauseated and vomits twice. He is admitted to the hospital for pancreatitis. Ned now wants to know how in the heck he got pancreatitis.

THE SUSPECTS

The likely suspects are the following drugs.

1. Alcohol (Ethyl Alcohol)

Alcohol is a recreational drink. It can cause intoxication resulting in abdominal pain, vomiting, blurred vision, or mental changes.[35] When asked about their consumption of alcohol, the majority of people underestimated the amount actually consumed.[36] In 2004 61 percent of adults in the United States drank alcohol; 32 percent of those who drank reported drinking at least five drinks on at least one day over the year.[37] Alcohol is one of the main causes of pancreatitis.

2. Tramadol (Trade Name: Ultram)

Tramadol is used to relieve moderate to severe pain. It can cause dizziness (33 percent), headache (32 percent), drowsiness (25 percent), insomnia (11 percent), flushing (16 percent), itching (12 percent), constipation (46 percent), or nausea (40 percent). Tramadol should not be taken with alcohol due to increased sedative effects.[38]

3. Losartan (Trade Name: Cozaar)

Losartan is used to treat high blood pressure. It can cause fatigue (14 percent), diarrhea (15 percent), urinary tract infection (16 percent), anemia (14 percent), or abdominal pain (4 percent). Losartan is in the drug class titled angiotensin receptor blockers (ARBs). ARBs also work to inhibit the action of angiotensin. A black box warning states that pregnant women should avoid this drug. Like ACE inhibitors, ARBs can also be harmful to a developing fetus. This medication should be stopped as soon as pregnancy is detected.[39]

LET'S RECAP

Patient: Ned, age 71
1. Alcohol: 2–3 beers a day
2. Tramadol (Ultram) for pain: 50 mg every 4–6 hours as needed for pain
3. Losartan (Cozaar) for high blood pressure: 50 mg daily
Lab-test results: All within normal limits
X-ray findings: CAT scan showing enlarged liver

SUMMARY REPORT

An initial evaluation of the situation suggests that Ned's pancreatitis *is* causing the symptoms. The following information explains the situation:

- CAT scans and a cross-sectional X ray are done of Ned's abdomen. The pancreas is usually seen as a gray area that has a defined outline and is solid in appearance. Ned's CAT scan shows a diffuse, enlarged, and splotchy pancreas.

- The pancreas functions to secrete enzymes involved in digestion. In pancreatitis, the pancreas is essentially being eaten away by these enzymes, which explains its appearance.

The Culprit: The Abuse of Alcohol

Prolonged alcohol use is to blame for 70 percent of chronic pancreatitis cases and 35 percent of acute pancreatitis cases, making it the second-most-common cause of pancreatitis behind gallstone obstruction.[40] The mechanism of alcohol-induced pancreatitis is also unclear, although hypotheses suggest that long-term use of alcohol alters the pancreatic fluid and promotes blockage of the pancreatic ductules.[41] Case reports have suggested that losartan and other ARBs (such as Atacand, Avalide, Diovan, and Micardis) are associated with inducing pancreatitis, although the mechanism by which they do this is not understood.[42] Losartan has been loosely associated with pancreatitis by case reports, but the association has never been definitively proven in any clinical trials. Therefore, losartan cannot be blamed as the cause of Ned's pancreatitis. Losartan gets off the hook for this one.

THE SOLUTION

Ned is kept in the hospital, where he is given fluids, pain medicine, and drugs for nausea. Because the pancreas helps make enzymes to digest food, he is restricted from food for a couple of days and given calories through his IV (also known as a TPN, or total parenteral nutrition). He is also given antibiotics to minimize the risk of infection around the pancreas. Ned's health-care provider explains how alcohol caused his pancreatitis and that Ned needs to cut down his drinking to one or two glasses a week.

WHAT ARE YOUR CHANCES?

Acute pancreatitis caused solely by drugs is considered very rare, amounting to approximately 1.4 percent of acute pancreatitis cases.[43] Although it can't be proven, Ned's losartan use may have contributed to his pancreatitis. About forty cases of pancreatitis occur for every one hundred thousand people each year.[44] This means that approximately 120,000 cases of acute pancreatitis occur in the United States annually, with only 1,700 caused by drugs. Alcohol is by far the biggest contributor to pancreatitis, at 70 to 80 percent of all cases. In 1999 pancreatitis accounted for 3,289 deaths; acute pancreatitis accounted for 84 percent of those deaths.[45]

HELPFUL ADVICE

The risk of developing pancreatitis from these medications is extremely rare. The average patient on therapy with losartan and hydrochlorothiazide should not worry about developing this complication from therapy; however, when alcohol is introduced, the risk of pancreatitis dramatically increases. The patient should recognize that alcohol is a drug and can have some additive adverse effects when combined with other drugs. Following Rule #10 in the future should help eliminate the risk of recurrence.

Even though it is rare for just one drug to cause pancreatitis, unless it is a high dose, keep in mind that other factors may contribute to developing the condition, such as alcoholism (or excessive and prolonged alcohol use) and other diseases. If you are taking drugs associated with pancreatitis, seek medical attention if you experience nausea, severe abdominal pain, or vomiting. Discontinuing the drug associated with pancreatitis may be warranted. Many factors can cause abdominal pain, and laboratory and radiology tests can determine whether pancreatitis is indeed the issue. Some risk factors for pancreatitis include high calcium levels; immunosuppression; autoimmune disease, such as Crohn's; and high fat levels.[46]

Not all problems have a simple culprit. Some drug-related problems may lead to the need for other drugs, which, of course, increases your risk for even more drug-related problems.

A couple of medications can increase the risk of pancreatitis. Pancreatitis caused by drugs accounts for about 5 percent of all pancreatitis cases. The following drugs are known to cause pancreatitis: thiazides (furosemide, hydrochlorothiazide); pentamidine (Nebu-Pent); antibiotics, such as tetracyclines and sulfonamides; valproic acid (Depakote); estrogens; and medications that suppress the immune system, such as azathioprine and 6-mercaptopurine. Some other medications may be associated with an increased risk, such as corticosteroids (Sterapred, Deltasone), NSAIDs (Motrin, Advil), acetaminophen (Tylenol), erythromycin, methyldopa (Aldomet), metronidazole (Flagyl), nitrofurantoin (Furadantin), ACE inhibitors (lisinopril, enalapril), and aspirin. Other risk factors include chronic alcohol use, African-American ethnicity, gallbladder disease, cystic fibrosis, and being male. If you are taking any of these medications or have any of these risk factors, see your doctor if you experience any of the following symptoms: nausea and vomiting, an intense and persistently swollen/tender abdomen, oily stools, or unexplained weight loss.

To help prevent pancreatitis, avoid excessive alcohol consumption, stop smoking, avoid a high-fat diet, eat smaller meals that contain more carbohydrates, and drink plenty of fluids.[47]

VIOLATION OF RULE #10: Understand That Over-the-Counter Medicines, Herbals, and Alcohol Are All Drugs

Ned thinks that alcohol can't cause medical problems, such as his pancreatitis. Boy, is he wrong. Patients who chronically consume alcohol should be aware of the serious health risks associated with the use of this drug. Alcohol affects many organ systems in the body. Those organs most commonly affected include the liver, gastrointestinal tract, heart, neurological system, and pancreas. Alcohol can also contribute to cancer. In addition, alcohol alters mental status, so if you are going to drink alcohol, drink responsibly. At most, men should drink two drinks per day, and women should drink one drink per day. A drink is considered a 12-ounce beer, a 4-ounce glass of wine, or 1.5 ounces of 80-proof liquor. Stick to the recommended amount to avoid long-term health consequences, such as pancreatitis.

CONDITION

Medication-Induced Diabetic Complications

The following case shows us that some medications can increase the complications of diabetes. Diabetic complications can include low blood sugar or high blood sugar.

THE PATIENT

Kristi Jo is an independent sixty-seven-year-old woman. She hates to ask for help with anything, but Kristi Jo is not in the best of health. High blood pressure and insomnia have always plagued her. She was also diagnosed with type 2 diabetes a few years back, and, according to her doctor, she has a hard time controlling her blood sugar levels. Kristi Jo has always said she feels fine and doesn't need the doctor's help. She rarely goes to the lab for the tests the doctor orders. Kristi Jo does visit him regularly, because she has trouble with frequent, painful bathroom trips. Her doctor tells her to control her blood sugar to make these episodes stop. Kristi Jo asks him to give her refills on the antibiotic (nitrofurantoin) she takes for recurring urinary tract infections so she doesn't have come back to him so often. The doctor reluctantly does what she says.

THE SYMPTOMS

Recently, Kristi Jo has had very high readings on her home blood sugar machine. She decides to double the dose of medication the doctor gave her. In her mind, she needs to cut her readings in half, so why not double her dose? A few days later, she is constantly feeling confused and anxious. Then one morning her neighbor comes over and finds her on the floor and immediately calls for an ambulance.

THE SUSPECTS

The likely suspects are the following drugs.

1. Nitrofurantoin (Trade Name: Macrobid)

Nitrofurantoin is an antibiotic that kills bacteria, but it can also cause nausea (8 percent), headache (6 percent), gas/bloating, diarrhea, and upset stomach. Severe reactions to nitrofurantoin involving the lungs have been noted. These cases can be life-threatening but are considered extremely rare. Peripheral neuropathy, or numbness in fingers and toes, can occur on long-term therapy.[48]

2. Temazepam (Trade Name: Restoril)

Temazepam is used as a sleeping aid and can cause drowsiness (<10 percent), headache (<10 percent), dizziness (<10 percent), nervousness (<10 percent), and extreme fatigue (<10 percent). Pregnant women should not take temazepam. Other drugs similar to temazepam have been found to cause some fetal development problems. Never take temazepam with alcohol. The combination may have additive effects and cause severe sedation. Temazepam is associated with a next day "hangover."[49]

3. Glyburide (Trade Names: Diaßeta, Glynase, PresTab, Micronase)

Glyburide is used for the oral management of type 2 diabetes mellitus and works by stimulating insulin release (decreases blood sugar). Some of the reported reactions to glyburide include headache, dizziness, rash, nausea/vomiting, hypoglycemia (blood sugar too low), anemia, and heartburn. Hypoglycemia can occur with glyburide as well as with insulin regular (Humulin R), and the symptoms are the same.[50]

LET'S RECAP

Patient: Kristi Jo, age 67
1. Nitrofurantoin (Macrobid) for urinary tract infection: 100 mg
    2 times daily
2. Temazepam (Restoril) for insomnia: 15 mg at bedtime
3. Glyburide (Diaßeta) for diabetes, type 2: 10 mg 2 times daily
Lab-test results:
    Hgb A1C: 11.8 (normally <7)
    Blood sugar: 18 mg/dL (normally 90–130 mg/dL)
    BUN (blood urea nitrogen): 37 mg/dL (normally 7–18 mg/dL)
    SCr (serum creatinine): 3.2 mg/dL (normally 0.6–1.4 mg/dL)
Other tests:
    Urinalysis: positive (+) for white blood cells, positive (+) for bacteria

SUMMARY REPORT

An initial evaluation of the situation suggests that Kristi Jo's diabetes is not directly causing the symptoms and that the following information must be considered:

- Kristi Jo's Hgb A1C (a measurement of the amount of glycated hemoglobin in the blood; it measures blood sugar control over several months) is 11.8. This means her average blood sugar is extremely high (about 330 mg/dL). Compared to the normal range, this suggests her blood sugar levels fluctuate greatly. Ideally, they would remain relatively stable.

- When her blood sugar level is tested in the ambulance, it is 18 mg/dL (This is dangerously low; 90–130 mg/dL is the normal range). Low blood sugar can be a life-threatening condition.

- At the hospital, her kidney function tests indicate elevated levels. This means her kidneys are not functioning at a normal level. Her SCr is 3.2, and this level should normally be between 0.6 and 1.4.

- Urine tests show she still has the urinary tract infection (UTI), even after taking a full course of an antibiotic.

SOLVE THE MYSTERY

Kristi Jo has just recently developed feelings of confusion and anxiety, which are likely caused by low blood sugar. This usually means we can eliminate anything she has been taking long term, such as temazepam and glyburide. She was recently put on nitrofurantoin, which appears to be our prime suspect now. However, it looks like nitrofurantoin could not have committed the crime. After rechecking the facts, we can see that she has recently doubled the dose of glyburide, which is at the scene of the crime.

The Culprit: Glyburide

Glyburide increases insulin release, which ultimately decreases blood sugar. The reason Kristi Jo's sugar went so low was the result of two factors. First, she doubled her dose due to her high monitor readings. Glyburide cannot be given in response to high sugars. It is intended to be taken prior to a meal to help decrease blood sugar afterward. Doubling a dose does not mean blood sugar will be cut in half. Second, Kristi Jo's kidneys, which are responsible for removing the glyburide from the bloodstream, are not functioning well. This means she has more glyburide remaining in her system for longer periods of time. This circumstance, in addition to taking twice as much drug to begin with, assured that low blood sugars would certainly be the end result.[51]

Decreased kidney function is also a reason her antibiotics did not work. The drug needs to be filtered out of the blood and into the bladder, where the infection exists; however, her body could not do this, so the antibiotic was ineffective. Kristi Jo's doctor will have to choose an antibiotic that works with reduced kidney function.

THE SOLUTION

Due to her recent kidney tests, Kristi Jo is taken off the glyburide. Her kidneys cannot clear it efficiently enough for her to be able to use it effectively. She is switched to insulin to help better regulate her blood sugar. Kristi Jo also needs to check her blood more regularly so she can eat if her blood sugar level is low or take insulin if it is too high.

WHAT ARE YOUR CHANCES?

Hypoglycemia, or low blood sugar, is a common problem in the hospital setting. However, actual numbers largely go unreported to the FDA, because the cause is usually immediately known. (660,000 Rxs/12 Rxs per year for 1 patient = 55,000 patients × 16 percent hypoglycemia = 8,800 cases per year.) Only 23 glyburide patients were reported to the FDA in 2007 for having hypoglycemia.[52] Studies have confirmed the rate is low, but certain factors can increase a person's risk. Not eating after a dose of medication, taking too high of a dose, and decreased kidney function are all risk factors for hypoglycemia.[53]

HELPFUL ADVICE

Hypoglycemia is a common complication to diabetic therapy. The patient and family members should know the proper ways to diagnose and to treat an episode; however, following Rules #2 and #5 would have benefitted Kristi Jo, as mentioned earlier.

Never self-dose a medication if it does not seem to be working. This can be dangerous, as this case demonstrates. Kristi Jo's doctor or pharmacist should have informed her about how glyburide works. She chose to take her care into her own hands, and it nearly cost Kristi Jo her life. She needs to trust her doctor and her pharmacist, following their advice as well as the rules in this book. As for Kristi Jo's recurrent problems with UTIs, her blood sugar is the underlying problem. High glucose readings likely mean the urine contains glucose. This is the perfect food for bacteria and an ideal environment for bacteria to thrive in. Once her physician switches her to a different antibiotic, her UTI should be under control. Also, Kristi needs to practice better diabetic care. She should be testing her blood sugar a minimum of twice daily, and she should understand what to do to control hypoglycemia. She also needs to be aware of the long-term complications that come from poorly controlled diabetes, such as kidney problems, loss of vision, cardiovascular problems, and the possible need for amputation. She needs to take control of her diabetes and work harder to manage her diet and medications. Even though the risk may be low, when multiple factors combine, you may be the patient affected.[54]

VIOLATION OF RULE #2: *Know Your Kidney Lab Values*

Kristi Jo should have known her kidney lab values and understood more about her renal (kidney) function as well. Her glyburide reached levels that were too high because Kristi Jo's kidneys were not functioning as they should have been. With Kristi's diabetes and the medications she is on, her doctor should check Kristi's kidneys every three months. To control her diabetes, Kristi should check her blood sugar level twice daily (at a minimum), and have her HbA1C checked every three months to determine how well she is doing with her glucose control.

VIOLATION OF RULE #5: *Take Your Medications as Your Doctor Prescribed*

Kristi Jo broke one of the cardinal rules for the safe use of medications—she took it upon herself to adjust her meds without talking to her physician or pharmacist. Medications do not work the way most people think they do. They are very tricky, and only your doctor or pharmacist will know which dose is appropriate for you. Struggling with medication control for a disease can be very frustrating; however, it is important to remember that only a doctor should recommend any changes to your medication regimen. Stick to the prescribed regimen, and call or make an appointment to discuss any problems you may encounter with your medications.

CHAPTER 4

Are Your Meds Playing Tricks with Your Mind?

Medications are capable of producing many dangerous effects on the brain that can change a person's mental status. A change in mental status can cause confusion, memory loss, and reduced alertness. It is important not to underestimate the impact of medications on judgment, memory, mood, and manual dexterity.

CONDITION

Medication-Induced Psychosis — Case 1

The following case shows us that some medications can cause a psychosis, which is any severe mental disorder in which contact with reality is lost or becomes highly distorted.

THE PATIENT

Edna is everyone's favorite neighbor. She is seventy-eight years old and feels that it is her duty to be the neighborhood grandma. She always bakes goodies and gives out little knickknacks to the neighborhood kids. They all know where to go for the best chocolate-chip cookies in town! All the kids love her and think she is just the coolest old lady ever. But one day they find her wandering around outside in her pajamas, speaking gibberish. What in the world is wrong with Edna? Has she just lost it?

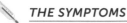

THE SYMPTOMS

One of the neighbors realizes Edna is not acting like herself and takes her to the emergency room. Edna complains of not being able to breathe very well, having an upset stomach, and being extremely tired all the time. The neighbor tells the doctor that Edna's mental state is usually very sharp. The doctor reviews Edna's medical background and determines she has previously been diagnosed with chronic obstructive pulmonary disease, depression, and seizures. She takes several medications to alleviate depression and to control her seizures. Her history includes a brain aneurysm (bleed) and smoking about one pack of cigarettes per day for more than fifty-five years. What has happened to this sweet old woman?

THE SUSPECTS

The likely suspects are the following drugs.

1. Phenytoin (Trade Name: Dilantin)

Phenytoin is used to treat and prevent seizures. The side effects include nausea, vomiting, dizziness, confusion, sleepiness, or gingival hyperplasia. Some changes in the body can affect phenytoin levels and cause any side effects to be more prominent. In 2006 phenytoin was one of the top two hundred most commonly prescribed drugs in the U.S. market.[1]

2. Mirtazapine (Trade Name: Remeron)

Mirtazapine is used to treat depression. It can cause sleepiness (54 percent), dry mouth (25 percent), increased appetite (17 percent), dizziness (7 percent), and abnormal thinking (3 percent). A black box warning states that mirtazapine may increase suicidal thoughts in children or adolescents (along with other antidepressants). This medication is taken at bedtime due to sedating side effects.

3. Duloxetine (Trade Name: Cymbalta)

Duloxetine is used for depression and nerve pain in diabetics. The side effects of duloxetine are sleepiness (21 percent), dizziness (17 percent), headache (15 percent), increased sweating (6 percent), nausea (38 percent), and dry mouth (15 percent). Duloxetine carries a black box warning stating that it may increase suicidal ideation (thoughts) in children or adolescents. In 2006 it was among the top seventy-five drugs most frequently prescribed in the United States.[2]

LET'S RECAP

Patient: Edna, age 78
1. Phenytoin (Dilantin) for seizures: 100 mg in the morning, 200 mg at noon, 200 mg at bedtime
2. Mirtazipine (Remeron) for depression: 15 mg at bedtime
3. Duloxetine (Cymbalta) for depression: 60 mg daily
Lab-test results:
   Phenytoin: 17 mcg/mL (normally 10–20 mcg/mL)
   Albumin: 1.2 g/dL (normally 3.4–5.4g/dL)
X-ray findings: Not applicable

SUMMARY REPORT

An initial evaluation of the situation suggests that Edna's chronic pulmonary obstruction and depression are not directly causing the symptoms and that the following information must be considered:

- Phenytoin concentrations in the blood must be monitored to make sure that the dose is not too high or low, because high levels can cause increased symptoms of lethargy and mental-status changes.

- Blood tests show that the amount of phenytoin Edna has in her body is 17 mcg/mL, which is in the desirable therapeutic range of between 10 and 20 mcg/mL. It is high enough to be effective but not so high as to be the likely cause of Edna's problems.

- Edna's albumin level is found to be very low at 1.2g/dL. This can become a problem when trying to measure the amount of active phenytoin in the blood, because a fraction of the phenytoin in the blood is bound to albumin.

SOLVE THE MYSTERY

Some of her other medications, such as phenytoin, mirtazepine, and duloxetine, can cause drowsiness, especially in the elderly. Mirtazepine is especially sedating, but it would not be causing the nausea and breathing troubles. Thus, we can rule out mirtazepine. Duloxetine can also cause sleepiness and a little nausea, but it is very unlikely that it would cause Edna to become this disoriented. Let's rule out duloxetine as well. We have a lot of information about the monitoring of phenytoin. Could it be the culprit?

The Culprit: Phenytoin (Dilantin)

Because phenytoin is highly protein-bound to albumin at more than 90 percent, anyone who is taking it must have their albumin levels monitored.[3] If the phenytoin molecule is bound to the albumin, it cannot leave the blood to move to its site of action—the brain. The portion of the drug that is *not* bound can pass through membranes to reach the brain where it works to combat seizure activity. If the blood contains a lower concentration of albumin than the amount needed for protein to bind, more of the phenytoin will be free and available to act on the brain. For example, if 90 percent of phenytoin binds to albumin, and the person has a phenytoin concentration of 15 mcg/mL with normal albumin, only 1.5 mcg/mL is able to reach the brain. But if the person doesn't have normal albumin, only 20 percent may be able to bind, so 12mcg/mL is able to reach the brain. Using a formula to correct for albumin, Edna's concentration was about 50mg/dL, which is far out of range.

THE SOLUTION

Edna is taken off the phenytoin (Dilantin) for a couple days to let it

clear from her body. When the corrected concentration of phenytoin returns to a normal amount, her health-care provider restarts
the phenytoin at a lower dose. She is brought back to the doctor's
office for lab tests over the next couple of weeks to make sure that
the corrected concentration is not too high.

WHAT ARE YOUR CHANCES?

In patients with lower albumin, a lower dose of phenytoin should
be used. The 2003 Annual Report of the American Association
of Poison Control Centers' Toxic Exposure Surveillance System
(AAPCC TESS) reported 2,173 unintentional phenytoin toxicities
in the United States, which resulted in 98 major morbidities and
10 deaths.[4] Extrapolation from more than five thousand urban
hospitals in one study shows that more than twenty-five thousand
patients are presenting with phenytoin toxicities in the emergency
department.[5] No reported incidence of phenytoin toxicity could be
located, such as ataxia (loss of balance), vertigo, or slurred speech
due to overdose. According to the FDA's MedWatch database,
twenty-eight reports of dizziness, ataxia, vertigo, mental status
changes, and falls were attributed to phenytoin.[6]

Your chances of developing phenytoin toxicity may increase if
you have a poor diet.[7] Your albumin level is a reflection of adequate
nutrition, and if you aren't eating enough, your albumin may go
down, thus increasing your chances for phenytoin toxicity.

HELPFUL ADVICE

This particular adverse effect from phenytoin therapy may not be
as common as some other possible complications. However, any
time the mental status of a patient changes, it is an extremely serious problem. This toxicity could be common if a patient fails to
have scheduled blood tests to evaluate phenytoin blood levels. Phenytoin has some unique characteristics that make dosing very tricky
for your doctor. Its dose-to-effect ratio is different from that of a
standard blood pressure drug. Overdoses are a distinct possibility,

because there is a fine line between the therapeutic, or desired, effect and the toxic effects Edna was experiencing. Other issues, such as malnutrition, vastly increase the risk of this toxicity. For future reference, Edna should know about Rules #4 and #6 to prevent this from occurring again. Phenytoin levels should be tested on a regular basis to make sure the proper dose is being administered. Edna's age means she is more likely to suffer from an episode like this one. Increasing the frequency of her monitoring should take care of this problem for good.

To avoid potential toxicity, people taking phenytoin should monitor the number and severity of their seizures and be aware of the signs and symptoms of toxicity: nystagmus (involuntary movement of the eyeball from side to side), decreased coordination, altered gait (difficulty walking), slurred speech, nausea and vomiting, confusion, and/or lethargy (abnormal drowsiness). If any of these symptoms are experienced, contact a doctor immediately. Low albumin increases phenytoin toxicity, and extremely high phenytoin levels can lead to coma, seizures, and possibly death.

If you are taking a drug that requires monitoring with blood labs, don't disregard them. Other drugs may also change concentrations of this drug, so it is important for any health-care provider prescribing new medications to know everything you are taking. The normal levels of phenytoin are 10 to 20 mcg/mL, and toxicities can be seen at any levels above this. I recommend that phenytoin levels be tested every six months.

Some medications can increase the levels of phenytoin and should be avoided; alternatively, your phenytoin dose can be adjusted accordingly. These medications include amiodarone (Cordarone, Pacerone); ethosuximide (Zarontin); fluconazole (Diflucan); valproic acid (Depakene); and oral anticoagulants, such as warfarin (Coumadin).[8] Talk to your doctor or pharmacist before starting any of these drugs, because they might increase your phenytoin levels and cause toxicities.

VIOLATION OF RULE #4: Be Aware That Elderly Patients Are Different from Younger People

This problem starts with Edna's being older. If Edna's physician had realized that Edna, along with many elderly patients, may have a reduced amount of albumin, this problem could have been avoided. She likely does not eat as much protein in her diet and therefore has a reduced albumin level. If you are an older patient, remind yourself and your doctor that medications can and do behave differently in the elderly. Make sure that your physician verifies that the prescribed use, dose, and indication are correct for someone your age.

VIOLATION OF RULE #6: Know Your Lab-Test Schedule

Had Edna been vigilant with her lab-test schedule, which includes a test for albumin, she and her doctor would have detected this problem earlier. If you are on phenytoin, you should have your albumin along with phenytoin levels checked at the beginning of therapy, and then again after any dosage changes (both increases and decreases); if seizures are controlled, check levels every six months just to make sure the phenytoin level is therapeutic but not toxic. A liver function test should also be performed before you start therapy and then repeated every six months. The liver metabolizes and excretes phenytoin. If your liver is not working properly, this toxicity could occur.

VIOLATION OF RULE #12: Know That Most Adverse Drug Reactions Are Due to Dosage Issues

If you notice any mental-status changes, double vision, slurred speech, loss of balance, or dizziness, it may be a sign that the dose you have been prescribed is too high. Contact your doctor or pharmacist immediately.

■■■■■ **CONDITION** ■■■■■

Medication-Induced Psychosis — Case 2

*The following case is another example of how a
medication can cause psychosis, regardless of the
patient's age.*

THE PATIENT

Zach is your average eighteen-year-old boy. He spends most of his time at home watching TV, playing video games, and doing homework. He would like to spend more time outside playing sports with his friends, but his asthma limits his activity most days. He also started smoking a few years ago and guesses that he smokes about one pack per day.

THE SYMPTOMS

Recently, Zach has had problems with his asthma and has been coughing up green mucus for more than one week. He starts having an asthma attack and is sent to the ER. He is admitted to the hospital and treated for bronchitis. He is started on prednisone to help with the inflammation and to allow him to breathe easier. After a day in the hospital, he starts to experience weird mental problems. He starts losing touch with reality and begins seeing things that aren't really there. He is becoming uneasy, anxious, and irritable. He is beginning to think he is going crazy.

THE SUSPECTS

The likely suspects are the following drugs.

1. Albuterol (Trade Names: Proventil, Ventolin)

Albuterol helps relieve the symptoms of asthma by relaxing the muscles in the lungs. Some side effects of this medication are dizziness, headache, nausea, rapid heartbeat, trouble sleeping, tremors, and shakiness. It is used as a "rescue" inhaler when a person with asthma is having symptoms. Asthmatics should always have some type of inhaler, such as albuterol, for relief from their attacks.

2. Prednisone (Trade Names: Sterapred, Deltasone)

Prednisone reduces inflammation for many different diseases. Some side effects include nausea and vomiting, upset stomach, appetite change, edema, headache, insomnia, anxiety, and mood swings.[9] Prednisone is widely used for many reasons and can cause immune suppression after long-term use. About 27.6 percent of patients will have some type of mental changes when taking higher doses.[10]

3. Nicotine (Cigarettes)

Zach recreationally uses nicotine in the form of cigarettes. The negative effects of cigarettes are taste changes, upset stomach, high blood pressure, rapid heartbeat, and bronchitis.[11] Approximately 20.6 percent of the U.S. population smoked cigarettes in 2005.[12] Tobacco smoke is noxious to the lungs and causes chronic inflammation, damaging the tissue and narrowing the airways. Airflow becomes restricted, and breathing becomes more difficult.

LET'S RECAP

Patient: Zach, age 18
1. Albuterol (Proventil, Ventolin) for Asthma: 1 or 2 puffs as needed every 4–6 hours
2. Prednisone (Deltasone) for severe asthma: 40 mg every 12 hours
3. Nicotine: 1 pack of cigarettes per day
Lab-test results: All within normal limits
X-ray findings: Not applicable

SUMMARY REPORT

An initial evaluation of the situation suggests that Zach's existing health problems are not directly causing the symptoms. Albuterol may cause anxiety and nervousness but not hallucinations.

SOLVE THE MYSTERY

Do you know what did it? Some people might say that smokers are foolish, because they continue to smoke even though they know it can cause cancer, but smoking cigarettes certainly doesn't make people see things! Albuterol might cause Zach to be restless, shaky, or anxious, but, once again, it wouldn't make him see things crawling on the walls. What else is left?

The Culprit: Prednisone

Prednisone, like any of the glucocorticoids, can cause psychological changes in almost one-third of people but usually manifests as mood changes and insomnia. Cases of prednisone's causing hallucinations are rare. Other psychological changes that prednisone can cause include depression, anxiety, insomnia, agitation, memory impairment, and delusions.[13]

THE SOLUTION

Zach is given a medicine to calm him down, and his doctor starts decreasing the dose of his prednisone, which needs to be stopped slowly to keep his asthma from becoming a problem again.

WHAT ARE YOUR CHANCES?

For most patients who are taking a high dose of prednisone, the chance of having problems like Zach's are between 3 and 6 percent.[14] The incidence of severe psychiatric syndrome in more than 2,500 patients is approximately 5.7 percent. Women are twice as likely as men to acquire steroid psychosis, but if you account for the higher incidence of women taking steroids, female predominance is only slight. If psychosis is going to occur, symptoms usually appear within the first six days, and the onset is usually acute. Even if someone has taken this medication before, they still run the same risk for developing this adverse reaction. In a review of literature, about 20 percent of patients who had steroid psychosis had a history of previous psychiatric disorders.[15] Prior mental disorders do not necessarily predispose you to the risk of this psychosis, but having a clear history of mental disorders doesn't mean this syndrome won't occur. In 2007 twenty-three million prescriptions for prednisone were filled. If we even assume that every patient was on chronic steroid therapy, which the vast majority was not, then 57,500 to 115,000 patients would be affected each year. (23,000,000 Rxs/12 Rxs per year for 1 patient = 1,916,667 patients × 3–6 percent incidence = 57,500–115,000 cases/year.) Only one case of hallucination was reported to the FDA's MedWatch system for 2007.[16] As previously stated, a reaction to prednisone leading to hallucinations and the prominent mental changes that Zach experienced are extremely rare. However, these reactions can be recognized and reversed if patients inform their physicians and pharmacists of any unusual side effects they experience when starting new medications.

HELPFUL ADVICE

This possible complication should not worry you when taking corticosteroids. Even if it does occur, the usual course of therapy is short, and symptoms will quickly resolve. Most problems occur with long-term corticosteroid therapy, and you should follow up on severe cases with a physician, because unpredictable mood swings can be troublesome to family members. Overall, about 40 percent of patients present with depression, 25 percent with mania (symptoms include rapidly changing behavior, decreased sleep, exaggeration), 5 percent with bipolar disorder (alternating mania and depression), 15 percent with agitated schizophrenia/paranoid psychosis (withdrawal from reality, delusions, hallucinations), and 10 percent with fast-onset delirium (mental confusion). The complete recovery rate from steroid psychosis is 90 percent, but 5 to 7 percent will have ongoing problems, and 3 percent commit suicide. It is important to notice symptoms as soon as possible so you can obtain help to prevent serious consequences.[17]

The dose and type of steroid plays an important part in the incidence of this steroid psychosis. The three most common corticosteroids that contribute to this condition are ACTH (adrenocorticotropic hormone), cortisone, and prednisone, but all corticosteroids have some potential to induce psychosis.[18] In the Boston

Collaborative Drug Surveillance Study, 1.3 percent of patients who were on fewer than 60 mg/day of prednisone showed psychotic symptoms, while patients who were on between 41 and 80 mg/day had a rate of 4.6 percent. If patients were on more than 80 mg/day, this rate went up to 18.4 percent, and the average daily dose where psychosis presented was 59.5 mg/day of prednisone.[19] The dosage does not appear to affect the onset.[20] Rule #11 for the safe use of medications could have helped in this case. This drug is unpredictable and affects different patients in different ways.

In this case, Zach experiences a form of psychosis while on prednisone. Certain risk factors may predispose someone to drug-induced psychosis, including being over forty, being an infant or child, high doses, altered liver/kidney function, and substance abuse, that may cause psychosis, head injury, and underlying disease states (lupus, Parkinson's, and HIV).[21] If corticosteroid therapy is needed, use the lowest dose possible, and discontinue as soon as possible. Look for signs or changes in the way you feel, and seek help as soon as you notice anything different. Patients who have been diagnosed with steroid-induced psychosis say they can feel the onset happening. Symptoms include increased irritability, swift changes in mood, anxiety, depression, unease, and oversensitivity to sound. Often, more serious symptoms will occur within seventy-two to ninety-six hours and can include distractibility, severe insomnia, extreme changes in mood, depression, confusion, auditory and visual hallucinations, agitation, memory impairment, and delusions.[22] Some side effects of medicines occur fairly quickly after starting the drugs. If you think that you are experiencing a side effect from this drug, call your health-care provider or pharmacist. If it is serious, seek emergency help immediately. The important thing is to notice any changes and to get help as soon as possible before full-blown psychosis takes place. Your doctor will be able to gradually reduce your steroid meds, if possible, or treat you with other medications. Explain the symptoms you are feeling to your doctor and why you think they may be related to your corticosteroid therapy.

VIOLATION OF RULE #11: If Your Health Changes after You Add a New Drug, Think Drug-Induced Disease

Some cases of drug-induced diseases are unpredictable and cannot be prevented. This is one such case. Zach took the prednisone to clear a case of bronchitis and to relieve his asthma symptoms. Unfortunately, changes in mental status for patients taking glucocorticoids can happen. The best thing Zach and his physician can do is recognize the fact that some patients may have a reaction to medications—albeit rarely. As a patient, if you are experiencing any unusual symptoms or side effects after you begin a medication, ask your doctor or pharmacist if it is usual or something to be concerned about.

CONDITION

Medication-Induced Falling

The following case shows us that some medications can cause falling. Falling as a result of taking various medications occurs when medications affect balance or make one drowsy.

 THE PATIENT

Lillian is a sixty-year-old woman who has never really had perfect health. She has a long history of neck and back surgeries, high blood pressure, low thyroid hormones (hypothyroid), pain in her hands and feet, and depression. She does her best to try to control her health by not drinking alcohol or smoking.

 THE SYMPTOMS

Lillian has never been a graceful person, but she thinks that she is more clumsy now than ever. She notices that she tends to fall randomly as a result of general disorientation, and she finds bruises resulting from these falls. One day after waking up on the floor and not remembering falling, she finally decides to take the symptoms seriously and talk to her doctor.

THE SUSPECTS

The likely suspects are the following drugs.

1. Zolpidem (Trade Name: Ambien)

Zolpidem is used as a sleep aid for insomnia, but it does not come without side effects. These include weakness, dizziness, and ataxia (difficulty keeping balance). It works by slowing down activity in the brain but does not usually last past the eight hours of recommended sleep. It has also received a lot of media coverage related to such activities as people eating and walking in their sleep. Lillian is taking the extended-release form to help it last through the night (zolpidem [Ambien CR] 12.5 mg) and is doubling the usual dose.[23]

2. Lorazepam (Trade Name: Ativan)

Lorazepam is usually prescribed for anxiety but may also be used as a sedative or to treat insomnia and nausea. It can cause dizziness and drowsiness (<10 percent of patients), vertigo or general unsteadiness, and depression (1–10 percent). Lorazepam is in the class of benzodiazepines, which may be addictive.

3. Carisoprodol (Trade Name: Soma)

Carisoprodol is a muscle relaxant used for sore muscles. It can cause hypotension (low blood pressure), poor muscle tone, syncope (passing out), dizziness, headache, agitation, and depression. Lillian does not take this all the time — only when her muscles feel really sore.

LET'S RECAP

Patient: Lillian, age 60
1. Zolpidem CR (Ambien & Ambien CR) for insomnia: 25 mg before bedtime
2. Lorazepam (Ativan) for anxiety: 1 mg 3 times a day as needed
3. Carisoprodol (Soma) as a muscle relaxant: 350 mg 4 times a day as needed for muscle pain

Lab-test results: all within normal limits
X-ray findings: bone fracture from a fall

SUMMARY REPORT

An initial evaluation of the situation suggests that Lillian's underlying health conditions are not directly causing the symptoms and that the following information must be considered:

- More than one drug is causing the problem.

- Lillian's blood pressure is stable when she stands up. If her blood pressure were low, she might fall (especially after standing up too quickly or bending over).

- She has a normal heart rhythm. The doctors tested Lillian's heart for arrhythmias, which are a common cause of people passing out due to the impaired blood flow.

- The only physical finding is a fracture on the X ray caused from the falls.

SOLVE THE MYSTERY

She is on three different medications that can cause her to be sleepy or drowsy. I'm not sure about you, but it makes me wonder two things:

1. Who is prescribing all these medications?

2. How does Lillian even get out of bed in the morning?

The Culprits: The Combination of Lorazepam, Zolpidem, and Carisoprodol

All three of these medications can cause occasional dizziness. Even though none of them causes a large percentage of people to feel dizzy, the combination of all of them makes the reaction more likely. Lorazepam has a 3.4 percent chance of causing unsteadiness and a 6.9 percent chance of dizziness. Zolpidem only has a 1 percent chance of causing dizziness, but this usually occurs during the daytime after a normal dose.[24]

Lorazepam and carisoprodol are both meant to be taken only when needed, but Lillian says she takes them most of the time. Considering she is doubling the normal dose of an extended-release zolpidem, it is probably lasting throughout the day and significantly increasing the dizziness she experiences.

THE SOLUTION

Lily has her medicines changed. Her zolpidem is changed to the usual dose, which is not extended release. The doctors change her lorazepam to a different medicine for anxiety that is not long-lasting.

WHAT ARE YOUR CHANCES?

Falls in the elderly are fairly common. About one-third of people over age sixty-five fall every year, and 10 to 20 percent of falls are medication related.[25] In 2004 about 1.8 million elderly people were treated for falls.[26] Even though Lillian is not over sixty-five, she has enough medicine affecting her balance to put her at an increased risk. The number of medications that people take is directly related to their fall risk. Several other components increase the risk of falls in the elderly, such as a lack of muscle tone, spinal problems, and drugs that decrease overall stability. It is estimated that medicines alone cause about 13 percent of falls.[27] That means there are approximately 234,000 falls from drugs. (1,800,000 falls × 13 percent caused by drugs = 234,000 cases of drug-induced falls.) Only twelve falls due to zolpidem were reported to the FDA MedWatch system over the first three quarters of 2007 and the last quarter of 2006.[28] However, when multiple medications that increase dizziness are added together, the combination can be disastrous.

HELPFUL ADVICE

Drug-induced falls are a serious matter, especially for the elderly. Those patients at risk should be closely monitored, because falling could cause a vast array of health issues and even lead to death. Lillian is on two medications that should be avoided in the elderly (lorazepam and carisoprodol) due to the increase in the risk of falls. Generally benzodiazepines should be avoided in the elderly, but if you must take a benzodiazepine, temazepam (Restoril), flurazepam (Dalmane), triazolam (Halcion), and estazolam (Prosom) are all short acting and may help decrease falls. These should be used at a lower dose in elderly patients.

Because of the potential severity of this issue, drug-induced falls should be considered one of the more dangerous yet widely unknown complications with prescription drugs. Rules #9, #12, and #15 should be followed here. Taking all these medications together should have raised the alarm for Lillian's pharmacist and may have prevented this fall. These medications are especially unpredictable in the elderly and should be prescribed with caution.

You have many ways to protect yourself from falls caused by your medications. The most common medications that increase the likelihood of falling include antidepressants, antipsychotics, and benzodiazepines. Drugs with anticholinergic effects (dry mouth, memory impairment, increased heart rate, constipation, blurred vision, or loss of coordination) are the worst offenders. Some drugs that have anticholinergic effects are tricyclic antidepressants, antihistamines, gastrointestinal antispasmodics, Parkinson's medications, and medications for urinary incontinence. Following is a more detailed list of medications that are known to increase the risk of falls.[29]

Medications Known to Increase the Risk of Falls

Class of Drug	Drug Names
Alcohol-containing medications or beverages	Cough medicines, Nyquil
Antiallergy medications (sedating antihistamines)	Benadryl, Unisom
Antianxiety medications (Anxiolytics)	Atarax, Ativan, Buspar, Tranxene, Valium, Vistaril, Xanax
Antidepressant medications (tricyclic antidepressants)	Elavil, Norpramin, Pamelor, Sinequan, Tofranil, Vivactil

(cont'd.)

Medications Known to Increase the Risk of Falls (cont'd.)

Class of Drug	Drug Names
Antiseizure medications (anticonvulsants)	Depakene, Depakote, Dilantin, Felbatol, Neurontin, Tegretol, Zarontin
Gastrointestinal-antispas-modic medications	Bentyl, Donnatal, Levsin, Librax, Pro-Banthine, Reglan, Scopolamine
High-blood-pressure medications/cardiovascular agents	Accupril, Adalat, Calan, Capoten, Cardi-zem, Catapres, Inderal, Isoptin, Monopril, Nitro-Dur, Prinivil, Procardia, Tenormin, Vasotec, Verelan
Hypoglycemic medications	Diaßeta, Glucophage, Insulin, Micronase
Overactive-bladder medica-tions	Detrol, Ditropan
Pain medications/skeletal-muscle relaxers	Flexeril, Lortab, Roxanol, Skelaxin, Tylenol with Codeine, Vicodin
Parkinson's medications	Artane, Azilect, Mirapex, Neupro, Parlodel, Requip, Trihexane
Sleep medications (sedative hypnotics)	Dalmane, Nembutal, Restoril, Seconal
Tranquilizer medications (Psychotropics)	Clozaril, Compazine, Haldol, Loxitane, Mellaril, Navane, Prolixin, Risperdal, Stelazine, Thorazine, Trilafon
Water-retention medications (diuretics)	Demadex, Dyazide, Lasix, HydroDiuril, Maxzide, Zaroxolyn

These medications should be avoided if a patient is at risk for falls. If a drug must be taken, use it at the lowest dose for the shortest amount of time. This list is not all inclusive but is meant to help you identify types of drugs that may increase the risk of falling.

Some basic tips will help you avoid falls while on any of these medications: Take your time with tasks, go to the bathroom before going to bed, avoid alcoholic beverages, exercise regularly, make your home safe (by adding more lighting, clearing up clutter, placing things within reach, and installing hand rails and antislip mats in the bathtub), check your vision, and get checked for osteoporosis.[30]

Also, have your doctor or pharmacist assess the need for all your medications and make sure that you are using the lowest effective dose or increasing the dosage slowly.[31]

If you find yourself having problems with falling, alert your doctor immediately. Also, look for trends in these symptoms, and try to avoid them. For example, if you start taking a medication that is known to cause dizziness, pay attention and note whether you stub your toe more frequently after beginning this new drug. It may be necessary to discontinue one or more of the drugs that are causing the problem, especially if you are elderly or have osteoporosis or an increased risk for getting broken bones.

■ CONDITION ■

Medication-Induced
Serotonin Syndrome

Serotonin is a neurotransmitter that helps regulate numerous bodily functions. The following case shows us that some medications can cause serotonin syndrome, a condition that occurs when medications cause high levels of the serotonin to accumulate in the body.

THE PATIENT

Georgia has been a stay-at-home wife and mom for almost her whole adult life. She was diagnosed with bipolar disorder at age twenty. Her condition interfered with her life so much that she was unable to work, so she took on the role of full-time mom. Most of the time, Georgia is a very loving and mellow person, but when she becomes sick, it is a different story. Her bipolar disorder gives her episodes of sleepless nights and causes her to start lots of activities that she may not finish or to do them over and over (mania).

These episodes are generally followed by episodes of the blues (depression). Last week Georgia went to the doctor because she felt very sad, and this feeling came on for no apparent reason. The doctor gave her a new medication called Lexapro (escitalopram) and wished her luck.

THE SYMPTOMS

Georgia has become very confused over the past couple of days, so her loving husband takes her to the emergency room. Because Georgia seems disoriented, the doctor interviews her husband to determine what has been going on. Georgia's husband mentions that Georgia has shaky hands (clonic movements), stares off into space, and has been very confused. She has been sweating excessively and complaining of a racing heart. He also tells the doctor that Georgia has bipolar disorder, high blood pressure, and low thyroid hormone.

THE SUSPECTS

The likely suspects are the following drugs.

1. Escitalopram (Trade Name: Lexapro)

Escitalopram is used to treat depression. It can cause the following problems: headache (24 percent), insomnia (9–12 percent), nausea (15 percent), and dizziness/fatigue (5 percent). It belongs to a common class of antidepressants called selective serotonin reuptake inhibitors (SSRIs).[32] By stopping the reuptake of serotonin from the brain, it allows more serotonin to be present within the synapse and may help with disorders associated with a lower-than-needed concentration of serotonin. The use of this type of medication has increased over recent time. In 2006 Lexapro ranked ninth among the top two hundred dispensed drugs, with a total of 3.2 million prescriptions dispensed in the United States.[33] A black box warning on this medication states that it may increase suicidal thoughts in children and adolescents.

2. Levothyroxine (Trade Names: Synthroid, Levothroid, Levoxyl, Unithroid)

Levothyroxine is prescribed for patients whose bodies do not produce enough or cannot produce thyroid hormone (hypothyroid). The job of thyroid hormone is to regulate metabolism. Because levothyroxine is essentially the same as the hormone naturally produced by the body, the side effects are not lengthy unless a person is taking too much or too little of it. Physicians monitor this by checking a person's thyroid hormone concentration (T3, T4, and TSH). Side effects may include insomnia, fatigue, anxiety, and increased heart rate. It should also be noted that side effects experienced depend on whether the thyroid level is too high or too low.[34]

Disease of the thyroid affects millions of people in America. In fact, levothyroxine was one of the top ten most prescribed drugs in 2006, with 30,914 million prescriptions dispensed that year.[35] Additionally, women experience this deficit much more frequently than men. To absorb enough thyroid hormone into the system to maximize the benefits, the tablet must be taken in the morning at least thirty minutes before a meal.

3. Lithium (Trade Names: Eskalith, Lithobid)

Lithium helps patients who have a bipolar disorder, more specifically the manic phase of bipolar disorder. Lithium carbonate can cause tremors, nausea, excessive urination, and other annoyances. To assist a physician in prescribing lithium, blood concentrations are measured to make sure the dosage is correct and to prevent excess intake that could cause adverse side effects. The exact frequencies of these adverse effects are not defined and are dependent on the blood levels, but about 30 percent of patients are intolerant of lithium. The normal range for lithium blood level concentration is 0.6 to 1.2 mEq/L. Two of the side effects (hypothyroidism and a decrease in kidney function) can be monitored by simple blood tests.[36]

Approximately 5.7 million Americans older than eighteen have some degree of bipolar disorder. Bipolar disorder is the sixth leading cause of disability in the United States.[37] Lithium is commonly used in bipolar disease, either alone or in combination with other medications, although the exact number of prescriptions written for it each year is not obtainable.

LET'S RECAP

Patient: Georgia, age 56
1. Escitalopram (Lexapro): for depression: 10 mg daily
2. Levothyroxine (Synthroid) for low thyroid hormone: 150 mcg daily
3. Lithium (Eskalith or Lithobid) for bipolar disorder: 300 mg 3 times a day

Lab-test results:

    Lithium: 1.0 mEq/L (normally 0.8–1.2 mEq/L)

    SCr (serum creatinine): 0.4 mg/dL (normally 0.6–1.4 mg/dL)

    TSH (thyroid stimulating hormone): 0.95 (normally 0.5–4.7)

X-ray findings: Not applicable

SUMMARY REPORT

An initial evaluation of the situation suggests that Georgia's medical condition is not directly causing the symptoms and that the following information must be considered:

- According to the list of suspects, the doses of each medication are considered to be within normal limits.

- Georgia's levothyroxine can cause increased heart rate and sweating, but she has been stable on 150 mcg daily for quite some time and never had problems before.

- Two of the patient's medications are being used for psychiatric conditions.

- Evidence shows that lithium may have indirect effects on serotonin.

- Georgia's kidney function is normal.

- The lithium and thyroid blood values monitored by the doctor are normal.

- Escitalopram is the only new drug she is taking.

SOLVE THE MYSTERY

So let's piece this puzzle together. Levothyroxine is unlikely to be the culprit. So that leaves escitalopram and lithium. Could two suspects be involved in this crime of drug-induced disease?

The Culprits: Escitalopram and Lithium

The symptomatic evidence of confusion, the exhibition of clonic movements (shaky hands), the hypertension (increased blood pressure), the mild increase in temperature, the diaphoresis (increased sweating), and the tachycardia (increased heart rate) point us in the direction of serotonin syndrome.[38] The drugs mentioned immediately above work together against the victim. Lithium causes the nerve synapse (where one nerve ending meets the beginning of another nerve) to be more sensitive to serotonin, while the escitalopram causes more serotonin to be present in the synapse.[39] This leads to an excess of serotonin at the synapse, resulting in the problems Georgia is experiencing. Just because the lithium and escitalopram (Lexapro) work on her central nervous system doesn't mean that they don't affect her blood vessels and rest of her body.

Currently no tests exist to concretely diagnose serotonin syndrome. Diagnosis is based on a medical history and thorough physical exam. The patient's history is positive for use of drugs that work on the serotonergic system. It should be noted that serotonin syndrome can cause death if not treated.

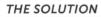

THE SOLUTION

If serotonin syndrome is suspected, the most effective way to resolve it is to stop the agents that are affecting the serotonin imbalance. Changes in vital signs are managed with supportive treatment that includes proper cardiac care, hydration, blood-pressure monitoring, and using measures to correct these imbalances. Georgia's well-being should return to normal as the drugs leave her body. A drug known as a benzodiazepine may be given to help with any muscle rigidity and spasms.[40]

WHAT ARE YOUR CHANCES?

Because it is increasingly common for a doctor to prescribe an agent that affects serotonin levels, the rate of occurrence for serotonin syndrome has increased. In 2004, according to the Toxic Exposure Surveillance System (TESS), 48,204 exposures to SSRIs (Escitalopram's class) resulted in mild to moderate outcomes in 8,187 patients and death in 103. Most deaths were a consequence of patients taking two agents that interacted or had similar activity.[41] Another source estimated that if a person is taking two different agents that modify the serotonin system, about 4 out of 1,000 patients will experience serotonin syndrome.[42] This can be estimated as 1 person in 250.[43] Only one case of serotonin syndrome was reported to the FDA's MedWatch system in 2007 in patients taking escitalopram (Lexapro).[44] This is likely because most cases are due to patients being on multiple medications that have serotonergic activity, making the numbers specifically related to escitalopram (Lexapro) difficult to interpret.

HELPFUL ADVICE

In the brain, serotonin helps regulate your mood, behavior, attention, and temperature. It also helps regulate many other bodily functions, such as vasoconstriction (manages blood pressure) and digestion, and it also affects platelets in the blood (which allow blood to clot) and the bronchioles (the airways in your lungs). Serotonin syndrome is a serious condition that can be life-threatening. Serotonin syndrome usually presents as a changed mental status along with problems that are of grave concern if not recognized early. Many people are not aware of the possible complication that can arise from taking one of the many over-the-counter (OTC) drugs (such as St. John's wort) that can exacerbate the problem. However, even in people taking multiple drugs that increase serotonin activity, the risk of this complication is relatively low. If Georgia had followed Rule #9, she may have never developed this complication. Always make sure a medical professional screens your profile for drug interactions.[45]

Medications That Contribute to Serotonin Syndrome[46]

Class of Drug	Drug Names
Analgesics	Codeine, fentanyl (Duragesic, Fentora), meperidine (Demerol), tramadol (Ultram)
Antibiotics	Linezolid (Zyvox), ritonavir (Norvir)
Dopamine agonists	Amantadine (Symmetrel), bromocriptine (Parlodel), levodopa
Herbal drugs or dietary supplements	*Hypericum perforatum* (St. John's wort), Panax ginseng, tryptophan
Monoamine oxidase inhibitors	Isocarboxazid (Marplan), phenelzine (Nardil), tranylcypromine (Parnate)
Other antidepressants	Bupropion (Wellbutrin), nefazodone (Serzone), trazodone (Desyrel), venlafaxine (Effexor)
SSRIs (selective serotonin reuptake inhibitors)	Citalopram (Celexa), fluoxetine (Prozac), fluvoxamine (Luvox), paroxetine (Paxil), sertraline (Zoloft)
Street drugs	Amphetamines, cocaine, LSD
Tricyclic antidepressants	Amitriptyline (Elavil), clomipramine (Anafranil), desipramine (Norpramin), doxepin (Sinequan) imipramine (Tofranil), nortriptyline (Pamelor), protriptyline (Vivactil)
Other OTC medications	Dextromethorphan
Other medications	Buspirone (BuSpar), lithium

This list is not all inclusive but shows you some of the medications that may lead to serotonin syndrome. If you are taking any of these medications, make sure you know how to recognize the signs and symptoms of adverse reactions. Symptoms to monitor for are muscle spasms, shaking, shivering, sweating, and confusion.[47] If you begin to experience any of these symptoms, obtain help as soon as possible and be sure to tell your doctor you are on one of these medications. If you are already taking one medication on this list and your doctor wants to place you on another, discuss serotonin syndrome and consider other alternatives to those medications.

VIOLATION OF RULE #9: Be Aware of Drug Interactions

Had Georgia, along with her doctor and pharmacist, been aware of the risks associated with adding escitalopram (Lexapro) to her drug regimen, she may have prevented this hospitalization. Escitalopram (Lexapro) is known as an SSRI (selective serotonin reuptake inhibitor). Its drug class is a dead giveaway that it might affect the serotonin system. Paired with lithium, this combination proves to be a serious problem for Georgia. She is lucky, as she does not experience the severe effects of serotonin syndrome, which may include death due to cardiac problems. Many medications, including herbals, can alter the serotonin system. Had Georgia read up on her drug interactions, she may have caught this mistake. As far as monitoring, not much can be done except to prevent the dangerous combinations. Prevention and early detection are critical. Always ask your doctor and pharmacist whether a new medication interacts with any medications you are currently taking. Also, double-check before taking any herbal products. As a patient, call your doctor immediately if you notice any of the following symptoms from a new medication for depression or mood swings: change in mental status, increased heart rate, increased blood pressure, increased sweating, and increased temperature.

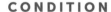 **CONDITION**

Medication-Induced Seizure

As the following case illustrates, medications can trigger seizures, which are episodes of abnormal electrical activity in the brain.

 THE PATIENT

Ruthie is a seventy-nine-year-old woman who spends most of her time taking care of her five cats and playing bingo at a local nursing home. Ruthie has one son who lives across the country in California. She sends lots of letters to her son and his children to keep in touch. She does not want to be part of the computer age, so she communicates in the old-fashioned way. Ruthie was diagnosed with a seizure disorder several years ago, and that condition has been controlled by the use of a couple of medications, until today.

THE SYMPTOMS

While in the middle of a game of bingo, Ruthie suddenly has staring spells and, subsequently, a seizure. When the seizure is over, she is very weak and confused. A fellow bingo buddy takes Ruthie to the emergency room. While in the hospital, she undergoes tests (including an EEG) to determine how her brain is functioning, but the doctor cannot conclude anything from these exams. An EEG, or electroencephalogram, measures brain waves and is commonly used to determine location and type of activity in the brain during a seizure. So what is going on with Ruthie?

THE SUSPECTS

The likely suspects are the following drugs.

1. Phenytoin (Trade Name: Dilantin)

Phenytoin is used for the treatment and prevention of seizures. It can also cause nausea, vomiting, dizziness, confusion, drowsiness, or gingival hyperplasia (excess growth of gum tissue). Some of these effects depend on the level of drug in the body.[48] In 2006 phenytoin was on the list of the top two hundred most commonly prescribed drugs in the U.S. market.[49]

2. Carbamazepine (Trade Names: Carbatrol, Tegretol, Tegretol XR)

Carbamazepine is used for the management of certain types of seizures, facial or jaw pain associated with a disorder called temporomandibular joint disorder (TMJ), and mania of bipolar disorder type 1. Side effects include dizziness (44 percent), drowsiness (32 percent), loss of balance (15 percent), nausea or vomiting, nystagmus (uncontrolled right to left movement of eye), confusion, elevated liver enzymes (AST [aspartate aminotransferase] and ALT [alanine transaminase]), and hyponatremia (low blood sodium concentration). Carbamazepine is a drug that requires blood monitoring to give the correct dose and to prevent toxicity. The reference range for the blood test is 4 to 12 mcg/mL. A reference range is the set of values of some measurement that a doctor uses to interpret the data from lab tests in prescribing a treatment for a patient.

This drug also carries a black box warning for causing severe abnormalities in blood cell counts and, in rare instances, a severe rash. A person should be aware of the early signs of these effects in order to catch them early. Doctors check patients' complete blood count (CBC) and platelet count (a blood test to measure the numbers and types of cells in your blood) to make sure no problem develops with their white blood cells. Possible effects include agranulocytosis, aplastic anemia, neutropenia, leukopenia, thrombocytopenia, pancytopenia, and anemia. These problems can have serious consequences in terms of how the blood cells function and protect the body. A doctor runs the blood tests mentioned above prior to treatment, then again at ten to sixteen weeks, then again at twelve months, and then every twelve months thereafter. Patients should have these required lab tests to make sure no serious problems arise from the use of carbamazepine.[50]

3. Ramipril (Trade Name: Altace)

Ramipril is used to treat high blood pressure. It is known to cause cough (7–12 percent), low blood pressure (11 percent), headache (1–5 percent), and high potassium levels (1–10 percent).[51] It is in the ever-popular class of antihypertensives called angiotensin-converting enzyme (ACE) inhibitors. As with other ACE inhibitors, ramipril (Altace) is commonly prescribed and was ranked forty-third out of the top two hundred drugs prescribed in 2006.[52] Ramipril also carries a black box warning about use in pregnancy, as ACE inhibitors can cause injury and death to a developing fetus when used in the second and third trimesters. Patients should discontinue ACE inhibitors as soon as pregnancy is detected.

LET'S RECAP

Patient: Ruthie, age 79

1. Phenytoin (Dilantin) for seizure disorder: 300 mg MWF, 200 mg TTSS
2. Carbamazepine (Carbatrol) for seizure disorder: 300 mg 3 times a day
3. Ramipril (Altace) for High blood: 5 mg daily

Lab-test results:

Carbamazepine: 14 mcg/mL (reference range normally 4–12 mcg/mL)
Phenytoin: 17.2 mcg/mL (reference range normally 10–20 mcg/mL)
Potassium (K): 3.7 mEq/L (therapeutic range normally 3.5–5.2 mEq/L)
Sodium (Na): 124 mEq/L (reference range normally 135–145 mEq/L)
X-ray findings: EEG: normal

 SUMMARY REPORT

An initial evaluation of the situation suggests that Ruthie's seizure disorder is not directly causing the symptoms and that the following information must be considered:

- According to the suspects list, the doses of each medication are considered to be within normal limits.

- The phenytoin level is therapeutic. The reference range for phenytoin is 10 to 20 mcg/mL.

- The carbamazepine level is 14 mcg/mL. The therapeutic range for carbamazepine is 4 to 12 mcg/mL.

- The one lab that is abnormal is the sodium. The reference range for sodium is 135 to 145 mEq/L.

- Ruthie's seizures are under control on her current regimen of anticonvulsants.

 SOLVE THE MYSTERY

Let's piece this together. Because this is a drug-induced disease reference, a drug must be causing this problem. The blood pressure medication is not known to induce seizures. Ruthie's phenytoin is therapeutic (at the proper level) and has been working. Her sodium is low, which can cause seizures, so which medication that she is taking can cause hyponatremia (a low sodium level)?

The Culprit: Carbamazepine

Lo and behold, Ruthie's lab value for carbamazepine came back somewhat high. Digging through the information on carbamazepine reveals that it is known to cause hyponatremia, or low sodium in the blood. Hyponatremia is a condition that occurs when the serum sodium level falls below 135 mEq/L. Nausea and weakness are usually the earliest symptoms, but the condition is generally asymptomatic. When symptoms do appear, the sodium concentration in the blood is frequently below 130 mEq/L. In the most severe cases, sodium levels are below 125 mEq/L, causing patients to experience headache, lethargy, seizures, coma, and respiratory distress.[53]

 ## THE SOLUTION

Ruthie is given IV fluids containing increased sodium to correct the imbalance. The sodium must be replaced at a slow rate to prevent other complications (brain swelling and additional nervous system problems). If she continues carbamazepine treatment, her sodium should be monitored closely in the future. Luckily, many other effective alternatives to carbamazepine are available for the treatment of seizure disorders, such as depakene and keppra.

 ## WHAT ARE YOUR CHANCES?

Approximately 2.5 million Americans have a seizure disorder. In addition, an estimated 10 percent of Americans will have a seizure at some point in time.[54] Hyponatremia associated with a treatment using carbamazepine is well known. It occurs in 1.8 to 40 percent of patients, varying with patient age.[55] In a study of patients with severe hyponatremia, 23 percent experienced a seizure.[56] Some risk factors have been identified that may increase your risk of developing hyponatremia in general. Risk factors include age (over forty), taking medications simultaneously that may cause hyponatremia (such as carbamazepine along with a diuretic or water pill), menstruation, psychiatric condition, surgery, and being female.[57] The exact incidence of a seizure of this type is unknown; even the FDA was unable to provide a figure. (2,070,000 Rxs/12 Rxs per year for 1 patient = 172,500 patients × 1.8–40 percent= 3,105–69,000 patients with hyponatremia.) Researching the FDA's MedWatch system reveals that carbamazepine was responsible for twenty reported cases of hyponatremia (low blood sodium) in 2007.[58]

HELPFUL ADVICE

Hyponatremia is a common complication of carbamazepine therapy. Treatment for hyponatremia depends on its cause. In this case, treatment involved adjusting Ruthie's dosage of the drug. Patients undergoing treatment with carbamazepine should be aware of the possible signs and symptoms of hyponatremia in order to reduce the risk of seizures. Although low sodium levels may be common to these patients, a seizure resulting from hyponatremia is less likely and mostly occurs in only severe cases, which would show signs prior to a seizure. Following Rule #6 may have prevented this seizure completely for Ruthie by detecting the low sodium level earlier.

Several drugs can cause hyponatremia, such as SSRIs and diuretics. Know which of your drugs can cause hyponatremia, and have your labs monitored as directed. Know the signs and symptoms of low sodium, especially if you are on a drug that decreases your sodium level. Signs and symptoms include headache, confusion, irritability, fatigue, seizure, and muscle cramps.[59]

Drug-induced seizures are often avoidable in general. Doses need to be adjusted for kidney and/or liver dysfunction. Avoid drugs with a potential to cause seizures, especially if you are at risk. Some risk factors include having a central nervous system (CNS) abnormality (infection, head trauma), being either an infant or elderly, having a history of seizures, kidney or liver dysfunction, metabolic abnormalities (causing changes in sodium, calcium, glucose, magnesium, phosphate, and albumin levels), rapid increases in doses, high concentrations of the drug, drug interactions, and fast administration of the drug. If you are starting a drug with a potential to cause seizures, such as anticonvulsants, lidocaine, procainamide, lithium, and theophylline, start at a low dose and increase it slowly. Serum concentrations of drugs need to be monitored.[60]

Several classes of drugs are known to cause seizures in elderly patients. Antipsychotics are one example. The risk of seizures increases if the person has a history of drug-induced seizures, an abnormal EEG (electroencephalogram), or a previous CNS complication or head trauma. Seizures usually occur when initiating an antipsychotic medication, or if the drug is used at higher doses or is increased at a fast rate. Clozapine and chlorpromazine carry the highest risk of seizures of all of the antipsychotics. Use a drug with a lower seizure potential if you are on an antipsychotic medication (such as risperidone). Antidepressants are another class known to cause seizures. Bupropion is an example of an antidepressant known to increase the risk of seizures and is contraindicated in patients known to have a history of seizures. Other examples of individual drugs are alcohol, insulin, isoniazid, lidocaine, theophylline, tramadol, and meperidine. With increasing age, many elderly individuals suffer from neurological disorders that place them at an increased risk of seizures, and risks increase further if the person has suffered cerebrovascular accidents or if they go to several different pharmacies to obtain their medications, which can lead to an increased risk of drug interactions.[61]

 VIOLATION OF RULE #6: Know Your Lab-Test Schedule

If Ruthie had gone in for her lab tests, this complication would have been noticed much earlier. If you are taking carbamazepine, prior to starting treatment you should have your complete blood count (CBC) tested with platelets and also have a liver function test, a urine analysis, and a check of your electrolytes (including sodium levels). The CBC with platelets should be checked again in ten to sixteen weeks after treatment begins, and then once a year to detect any decrease in the number of blood cells in the body caused by the carbamazepine. Have your urine analysis, concentration of carbamazepine, and electrolytes checked every six months to make sure your sodium level is normal.

████████ CONDITION ████████

Medication-Induced Digoxin Toxicity in Heart Patients

Digoxin is a medication prescribed to some patients who experience irregular heartbeats, including various forms of tachycardia. Unless dosages are tightly monitored, this drug can reach toxic levels within the body, as the following case indicates.

THE PATIENT

Larry is a sixty-seven-year-old retired truck driver. He was forced to retire about eight years ago, because his health started to decline. He loves the big open road and all the amazing sights he saw as he journeyed across the United States. Eight years ago Larry was diagnosed with the beginning stages of heart and kidney failure. He made a conscious decision to get out from behind the wheel of a big rig due to his health. About a week ago, Larry was put in the hospital for his heart failure. As with many people, upon being discharged from the hospital, Larry is starting on new medications.

THE SYMPTOMS

Larry's wife, Dolly, notices that Larry isn't eating much at any meals during the day. Dolly is a very good cook, and Larry usually loves just about everything she whips up in the kitchen. He complains of nausea, too. One thing that troubles Larry the most is that all lights have a greenish-yellow halo around them. Larry knows something is not right, so he asks Dolly to take him to the emergency room.

THE SUSPECTS

The likely suspects are the following drugs.

1. Furosemide (Trade Name: Lasix)

Diuretics are used to reduce swelling and fluid retention (edema) by excreting excess fluid via the kidneys. A diuretic can also treat high blood pressure by reducing fluid. This works by causing more salt and water to be eliminated through urine. Some side effects include frequent urination for up to six hours after taking a dose (which should decrease after taking furosemide for a few weeks), electrolyte imbalance, blurred vision, rash, and dizziness. Furosemide contains a sulfa compound, and some patients with sulfa allergies may have a reaction to furosemide. This medication comes in at number twenty on the list of the top two hundred products dispensed in the U.S. market in 2006, with 20,145,000 prescriptions.[62]

2. Digoxin (Trade Names: Digitek, Lanoxin, Lanoxicaps)

Digoxin is used for the treatment of congestive heart failure and to slow the ventricular rate in tachyarrhythmias (rapid, irregular heartbeats), such as atrial fibrillation, atrial flutter, and supraventricular tachycardia (cardiogenic shock). It essentially slows down the heart rate.

It also has negative effects that can cause "heart block" (a delay in the transmission of the electrical signals that cause the heart to beat), ventricular tachycardia or fibrillation, ST segment depression (changes on the EKG heart monitor), headache (3 percent), dizziness (5 percent), mental disturbances (4 percent), rash (2 percent), nausea, vomiting, diarrhea (2–3 percent), and some general weakness.

Digoxin is a medication that contains what is referred to as a narrow therapeutic index. This means that concentrations of this medication need to be maintained within a tight range. If the concentrations go above this range, which can happen easily because the range is so limited, a patient might experience digoxin toxicity. One noted side effect is hallucinations. The normal reference range for a digoxin blood test is arrhythmia 1.5 to 2.5 ng/mL and for heart failure 0.8 to 2 ng/mL.[63]

3. Isosorbide Mononitrate (Trade Names: Imdur, Ismo, Monoket)

Isosorbide mononitrate is used as a preventative treatment for chest pain. It helps dilate the blood vessels. It can cause headaches (19–38 percent), dizziness (3–5 percent), and nausea/vomiting (2–4 percent).[64]

Isosorbide mononitrate belongs to a class of medications known as nitrates and causes vasodilation (widening of blood vessels), which helps reduce chest pain. Some nitrates may also contribute to low blood pressure or worsening of heart failure. Some drug interactions are significant (involving the CYP3A4 enzyme), so patients should tell their doctors and pharmacists what other medications they are taking.

LET'S RECAP

Patient: Larry, age 67
1. Furosemide (Lasix) for fluid retention from congestive heart failure: 40 mg 2 times a day
2. Digoxin (Lanoxin) for heart failure: 250 mcg daily
3. Isosorbide mononitrate (Imdur) for vasodilator: 60 mg daily
Lab-test results:
　SCr: 2.4 mg/dL (normally 0.6–1.4 mg/dL)
　Digoxin: 2.2 ng/mL (normally 0.8–2.0 ng/mL)
X-ray findings: Consistently enlarged heart is shown on X ray

SUMMARY REPORT

An initial evaluation of the situation suggests that Larry's heart condition is not directly causing the symptoms and that the following information must be considered:

- Larry has been on furosemide since he was diagnosed eight years ago.

- Digoxin is a new drug added to Larry's regimen after his recent hospital admission for heart failure.

- Drugs should be prescribed cautiously because of Larry's impaired renal function. All of his medications are appropriate for his renal function except digoxin.

- Furosemide and isosorbide mononitrate's negative effects do not fit what is going on with Larry.

SOLVE THE MYSTERY

The previous clues are really leading to the conclusion that digoxin is causing this problem for Larry. Specifically, his blood level of digoxin is 2.2 ng/mL. What do you think? Which is the guilty party?

The Culprit: Digoxin

Nausea and vomiting, anorexia, visual disturbances, irregular pulse, and palpitations are good indicators that Larry is experiencing digoxin toxicity.[65] Other symptoms that may be present include overall swelling, difficulty breathing when lying down, impaired consciousness, decreased urine output, and excessive nighttime urination. Larry is seeing "halos," which is a hallmark indicator of digoxin toxicity. Larry is also not eating, a condition known as anorexia, another symptom of too much digoxin. Digoxin toxicity occurs when patients get too much digoxin in their systems and it accumulates, causing the symptoms just described. Larry's digoxin concentration is 2.2 ng/mL, as compared to the reference range of 0.8 to 2 for heart failure patients.

That doesn't seem too far out of range, right? Well, to complicate things even more, Larry has severely decreased kidney function. As you may have guessed, digoxin relies on good kidney function to remove the drug from the body. So Larry's body doesn't get rid of the digoxin as quickly or effectively as would a person with normal kidney function. Larry's digoxin dose should have been adjusted to account for his impaired kidney function.[66]

THE SOLUTION

The best solution for Larry is to stop his dose of digoxin and let the symptoms resolve. His heart should be monitored in case he starts to develop irregular heartbeats. Optimally, when the digoxin is restarted, his dose should be adjusted based on his kidney function to prevent another acute intoxication. For doctors, digoxin can be one of the trickier drugs to appropriately dose. If a physician is not careful, an overdose can happen. Larry's physician should monitor his electrolytes (serum potassium, magnesium, and calcium levels), because an imbalance here can cause more problems with digoxin use.

In severe cases of digoxin toxicity, an antidote-type drug is used, following the defined protocol for this type of medication. Also, depending on the severity of the toxic side effects, more supportive care measures and medications may needed (such as oxygen or antiarrhythmic drugs).[67]

WHAT ARE YOUR CHANCES?

One source estimates that as many as 1 to 5 percent of the population, or about three to fifteen million people, are on digoxin, and approximately 75 percent of these people are over age seventy-five. The actual incidence of digoxin toxicity is hard to define, because although a reported 35 percent of patients on digoxin are said to develop toxicity, many cases go unreported. The reported incidence in hospitalized patients is 15 to 20 percent.[68]

Approximately 0.4 percent of all hospital admissions are due to digoxin toxicity, and 1.1 percent of outpatients and 10 to 18 percent of nursing-home patients have also experienced this toxicity.[69] Certain people are at higher risk for digoxin toxicity than others, especially those with decreased renal (kidney) function, such as Larry. Other factors that can raise the risk for experiencing digoxin toxicity are increased age, heart failure, dehydration, low potassium or low magnesium levels, high calcium levels, and low thyroid hormone.[70] Another major contributor to digoxin toxicity is the long laundry list of its adverse drug interactions. It is extremely important that you, your doctor, and your pharmacist know every medication you are taking so that any potential interactions can be recognized before you start treatment. Therefore, depending on which medications you are taking, you may be at higher risk for this toxicity. (3,569,000 Rxs/12 Rxs per year for 1 patient = 297,417 × 35 percent incidence = 104,095 cases of digoxin toxicity/year.)

One retrospective study of multiple hospital admissions placed the overall incidence of digoxin toxicity as a diagnosis resulting in hospital admission at 4.8 percent of all patients taking this medication.[71] Locating information on digoxin toxicity as reported to the FDA MedWatch system is difficult. Digoxin toxicity presents as multiple symptoms and adverse reactions; however, in 2007 only seventy-four cases showed up in the FDA's MedWatch system as digoxin levels above therapeutic concentration, drug toxicity, or overdoses.[72]

HELPFUL ADVICE

Digoxin toxicity, as explained above, is common among those who take the medication. Considering the long duration of treatment, it seems many people will experience this complication at some point. Numerous adverse drug interactions are the key triggers for digoxin toxicity. When a new drug is added, the patient's digoxin level should be retested to screen for toxicity. For many patients, declining kidney function may also be one of the underlying causes of digoxin toxicity. Every patient on digoxin should have his or her digoxin levels checked frequently to decrease the high risk of this complication. Following Rules #1, #2, #6, and #11 could have prevented Larry's need for hospitalization.

With digoxin, it is especially important to make sure your doctor and your pharmacist know which drugs you are taking and to review them periodically with these professionals. Drugs that may increase digoxin levels include but are not limited to verapamil, quinidine, ritonavir, and amiodarone.[73] If you are prescribed one of these medications, tell your doctor to closely monitor your digoxin levels and to lower your digoxin dose, if necessary.

If you are elderly, you are more prone to digoxin's toxic effects due to the normal decline of kidney function. I recommend having your digoxin levels and kidney function evaluated every six months because of the risk of such toxicity.

Be aware of the signs of digoxin toxicity if you take the medication, including slowed heart rate (monitor pulse at home), nausea, vomiting, change in vision ("halos" around lights), dizziness, and confusion.[74] Digoxin is one of the worst offenders when it comes to

ER visits due to adverse drug reactions. Be informed of the side effects and toxicities associated with digoxin use, and go immediately to your hospital ER if you experience any of these effects. If you are elderly, make sure your physician has assessed your risk of falling. Digoxin use in the elderly has been associated with an increase in falls, which can lead to more complications.

VIOLATION OF RULE #1: Learn from Others—What Is Happening in the ER?

Larry and his doctor violated a number of rules. First, digoxin is one of the leading causes of hospital admissions and ER visits due to adverse drug reactions. Larry should have been more aware from the beginning of the complications related to digoxin use. Larry's doctor should have checked his digoxin levels within twelve to twenty-four hours if he gave him a "loading dose" (a dose of digoxin to bring the amount of drug in Larry's body up to a therapeutic level). If his doctor did not give a loading dose, the digoxin level should have been checked three to five days after Larry started taking the digoxin. Then, he should have checked the levels again five to seven days after any increase or decrease in dose. Digoxin levels should be checked at least once a year.

VIOLATION OF RULE #2: Know Your Kidney Lab Values

Larry's doctor should have also checked his renal (kidney) function and electrolytes (potassium, calcium, and magnesium levels), as they are very important in assessing digoxin toxicity. In Larry's case, not checking on his kidney's ability to function properly led to the overdose. Had Larry been vigilant with his monitoring and known his kidney lab values, this overdose could have been prevented.

VIOLATION OF RULE #11: If Your Health Changes after You Add a New Drug, Think Drug-Induced Disease

Larry also should have recognized that something just wasn't right when he started his multiple new drugs and should have asked his doctor for advice immediately.

Medication-Induced Hearing Loss

Your medication could affect your hearing. The following
case shows us that some medications can cause
hearing loss.

THE PATIENT

Sam is a forty-nine-year-old man who happens to be a huge audio-phile. He loves putting on an old album and kicking back while lis-tening to his favorite music. Pink Floyd's *The Wall* and their tune "Comfortably Numb" seem to be quite appropriate. He has a great love for his music and it really helps him relax, but Sam has had a few problems with his job lately. He stands for most of his shift and has suffered swelling in his legs at the end of the day. He is also bothered by arthritis in his knees. He has to put his feet up in the evening and loves to do so while listening to his music.

THE SYMPTOMS

Recently, Sam has had trouble hearing the high notes on his albums. Everything he hears sounds muddled and unclear. He calls his elec-tronics store, and a customer service rep takes a look at his stereo. The rep says everything is working just fine. Sam begs to differ. His wife thinks he is absolutely losing it. Sam decides to make an ap-pointment with his doctor to discuss the hearing loss, because it is quite disturbing. What could be going on with Sam and his hearing?

THE SUSPECTS

The likely suspects are the following drugs.

1. Celecoxib (Trade Name: Celebrex)

Celecoxib is a COX-II inhibitor that reduces inflammation caused by osteoarthritis. Side effects include hypertension (<13 percent), headache (10–16 percent), diarrhea (4–11 percent), skin rash (2 percent), edema/swelling (2 percent), dyspepsia (upset stomach;

9 percent), nausea, and abdominal pain (4–8 percent).[75] Rarely, severe gastrointestinal problems, including ulcers and GI (gastrointestinal) bleeding, are possible. Cardiovascular problems, including angina, stroke, and heart attack, are also possible. Patients should exercise caution if they have had serious GI problems or heart problems in the past. Celebrex (celecoxib) ranked thirty-fifth in total revenue generated by prescriptions in 2006.[76]

2. Furosemide (Trade Name: Lasix)

Furosemide is a diuretic used to reduce fluid retention or swelling (edema) and is also used to treat high blood pressure. It causes more salt and water to be eliminated via urine. Side effects include frequent urination for up to six hours after dose (although these effects should decrease after taking furosemide for a few weeks), electrolyte imbalance, blurred vision, rash, dizziness, and hearing loss.[77] Furosemide contains a sulfa compound, and some patients with sulfa allergies may have a reaction to furosemide. Furosemide came in at number twenty on the list of the top two hundred products dispensed in the U.S. market in 2006, with 20,145,000 prescriptions.[78]

3. Acetaminophen (Trade Name: Tylenol)

Acetaminophen is used for the treatment of pain, arthritis, muscle aches, and headache, and it is also a fever reducer. Side effects include rash, liver dysfunction (reduced liver function), and allergic reactions. All adverse reactions are rare, and acetaminophen is widely used without causing many serious problems. Acetaminophen use when combined with alcohol has the potential to cause serious damage to the liver; therefore, people with reduced liver function or damage should not use acetaminophen, nor should anyone drink alcohol while on acetaminophen. Acetaminophen is one of the most commonly recommended OTC medications for fever, arthritis, and pain by pharmacists and doctors.[79]

LET'S RECAP

Patient: Sam, age 49

1. Celecoxib (Celebrex) for arthritis/pain: 200 mg daily

2. Furosemide (Lasix) for swelling/edema: 40 mg every morning
3. Acetaminophen (Tylenol) for arthritis/pain: 500 mg 3–4 times daily
Lab-test results: All within normal range
Other tests: Bilateral hearing loss

SUMMARY REPORT

An initial evaluation of the situation suggests that Sam's arthritis and edema are not directly causing the symptoms and that the following information must be considered:

- Sam has started experiencing hearing loss over the last month or so after he complains about the swelling from being on his feet all day. His doctor prescribes furosemide (Lasix) to help control the swelling.

- Sam also says the acetaminophen (Tylenol) isn't cutting the pain, so his doctor prescribes celecoxib (Celebrex), which helps with his arthritis.

- Acetaminophen (Tylenol) has not been shown to have any effects on hearing loss.

SOLVE THE MYSTERY

Sam recently has started taking two new medications to combat the pain and swelling from his job-related conditions. He has recently started noticing problems with his hearing and is quite concerned. We can eliminate the acetaminophen, as it has not been reported to cause hearing loss. Two other suspects have long rap sheets for this offense, but which one could it be?

The Culprit: Furosemide (Trade Name: Lasix)

Furosemide is a type of diuretic called a "loop diuretic," and it helps reduce excess fluid in the body. People taking furosemide excrete more fluid to reduce swelling in the legs. This also helps in cases of high blood pressure and heart failure. In Sam's case, he is using the furosemide to eliminate excess fluid caused by being on his feet all day. He doesn't think his hearing loss could be caused by a drug.

Loop diuretics have the potential to cause hearing loss, or ototoxicity (damage to the inner ear caused by drugs or chemicals). Most commonly, this effect arises from the intravenous use of diuretics, but in Sam's case, it occurs with a standard dose that he is taking by mouth. Loop diuretics affect potassium levels in the body when they remove the excess fluid, because they also remove some of the extra potassium. Potassium is important for maintaining a gradient for nerves in the ear to transmit sound to the brain. If the potassium level is off even slightly, it can affect hearing.[80]

The Accomplice: Celecoxib (Trade Name: Celebrex)

Celecoxib may have contributed to Sam's hearing loss. Although specific data with celecoxib is limited, hearing impairment has been listed as a possible side effect. Patients should be aware that COX-II inhibitors, such as celecoxib (Celebrex), can cause hearing loss. Nonsteroidal anti-inflammatory drugs (NSAIDs), which work in a very similar fashion, have also been linked to hearing loss, so it is likely that COX-II inhibitors could be contributing to Sam's problem.

THE SOLUTION

Sam experiences some hearing loss once his doctor puts him on the furosemide and celecoxib. His doctor stops the furosemide and celecoxib, as they are the likely culprits. This time, Sam makes a full recovery, and his hearing returns. He is lucky, as he can now hear his albums just fine. His doctor increases his acetaminophen dose and suggests that Sam wear some support stockings to reduce the swelling in his legs during the day.

WHAT ARE YOUR CHANCES?

Hearing loss is a rare problem with most medications. With furosemide, most reported cases are caused by high IV doses. One source stated that 6 to 8 percent of patients taking loop diuretics could experience this adverse drug reaction. However, it was also reported that most are due to high IV doses in patients with renal failure. Rarely have patients taking furosemide orally reported hearing loss.[81] When looking at the number of patients affected, approximately one hundred thousand cases of ototoxicity due to furosemide could be possible in any given year. (20,145,000 Rxs per year/12 Rxs per year for 1 patient = 1,678,750 Rxs × 6–8 percent hearing loss = 100,725–134,300 patients experiencing hearing loss per year.) However, this number is likely grossly overestimated. Nearly all patients experiencing hearing loss with furosemide are on high-dose IV treatment. The FDA's MedWatch site listed two cases of ototoxicity due to furosemide in 2007.[82] No cases of celecoxib (Celebrex) causing hearing loss could be located in the literature.

HELPFUL ADVICE

As mentioned earlier, hearing loss is not a common adverse reaction with the use of oral furosemide treatment. Loop diuretics cause hearing loss at high doses and usually only when given intravenously. Hearing loss with furosemide is most likely to occur when furosemide is paired with another medication that also has the propensity to cause hearing loss. No one knows for sure how much higher the risk for hearing loss is when two ototoxic medications are paired together for treatment. Regardless, patients and family members should be aware of the possibility of such a reaction. Refer to the patient handouts, and ask your doctor or pharmacist for information about any side effects that you should know about. As always, if something changes with your health after adding a new medication, think drug-induced disease. Following Rule #11 could have helped Sam recognize this problem earlier.[83]

Hearing loss with oral loop diuretics is extremely rare, but you should be aware of this possibility. This means that if something with your body, such as your hearing, changes when a new medication is added, think drug-induced disease. Unfortunately, Sam is just an unlucky patient who happens to be a victim of an adverse reaction, but he recognized it early enough to seek help. Hearing loss can be irreversible if the furosemide is not stopped early enough. For a serious music fan, this would have been devastating.

Other medications that are known to cause hearing loss are included in the following chart. If you are taking one of these medications, be aware that they may alter your hearing. One easy way to determine hearing loss is to ask for a baseline hearing exam *before* you start any drug-related treatment. This will allow both you and your doctor to note any changes in your hearing.[84]

 VIOLATION OF RULE #11: *If Your Health Changes after You Add a New Drug, Think Drug-Induced Disease*

Had Sam been vigilant about any changes in his health, he may have noticed his hearing loss earlier. Sam is lucky, because his hearing returned. Some patients are not so lucky. Note any changes with the use of a new medication, as they can be a sign of an adverse reaction to the drug. Talk with your doctor and pharmacist about any unusual side effects once you start a new medication. These may be serious and are best resolved if caught early. Be aware of the drugs that can cause ototoxicity.

Ototoxic Medications That Can Damage Your Hearing[85]

The table below provides a list of medications that can adversely affect your hearing. Ask for a baseline hearing exam and have one performed periodically thereafter to make sure your hearing is not suffering due to a medication.

Medication Class	Drug Names/Examples
Aminoglycoside antibiotics	Amikacin, Gentamicin, Kanamycin, Neomycin, Streptomycin, Tobramycin
Antineoplastics (chemotherapy drugs)	Carboplatin, Cisplatin
Loop diuretics	Bumetanide, Ethacrynic Acid, Furosemide
NSAIDs	Diclofenac, Etodolac, Fenoprofen, Ibuprofen, Naproxen, Piroxicam, Sulindac
Quinine	Chloroquine, Quinine
Salicylates	Aspirin

CHAPTER 5

Are Your Meds Causing Bleeding Problems?

One of the most frightening adverse effects of medications is bleeding, including bleeding from the gums, blood in the urine and stool, and bruising. Bleeding can also occur in the brain, gastrointestinal tract, urinary tract, and abdomen.

CONDITION

Medication-Induced Subcutaneous Bleeding (Bruising)

The following case shows us that some medications can cause bruising.

THE PATIENT

Marty is a retired seventy-year-old man who enjoys spending time with his young grandchildren. He's had problems in the past with obesity, high cholesterol, and high blood pressure, as well as heart trouble. He has a heart condition known as atrial fibrillation (irregular heartbeat), so he has been taking Coumadin (warfarin) to prevent blood clots from forming (due to his atrial fibrillation) for the past couple of years. He knows he needs to exert better control over his diet and increase his activity level. He gets his international normalized ratio (INR) checked fairly regularly, but it is still fluctuating. The INR is a value that detects how well the blood is clotting. A higher INR means the blood is thinner, and bleeding is a risk with an INR higher than 3. Marty's INR level is shown to be a little low at his last doctor's appointment, so the doctor slightly increases his dose of warfarin for a couple of days each week.

THE SYMPTOMS

Marty has recently been noticing that he bruises more easily while playing with his grandchildren. He was playing baseball and pitching to the kids the other day, when one of them accidentally hit a line drive right back at his shin. He has since noticed that his entire lower leg has bruised and is now becoming a little swollen. He has also felt dizzy and nauseated during the past day or two since he was hit with the baseball. He has even vomited a couple of times. After he throws up, his nose starts bleeding. Marty thinks he might have just caught the flu and doesn't want to be a big wimp about his bruise. His wife expresses her concern and finally convinces her husband to go to the hospital.

THE SUSPECTS

The likely suspects are the following drugs.

1. Furosemide (Trade Name: Lasix)

Furosemide is a diuretic used to reduce fluid retention or swelling (edema) and also treats high blood pressure. It causes more salt and water to be eliminated via urine. Furosemide can cause frequent urination for up to six hours after a dose (this should decrease after taking furosemide for a few weeks), electrolyte imbalance, blurred vision, rash, and dizziness. It contains a sulfa compound, and some patients with sulfa allergies may have a reaction to furosemide.[1] Furosemide came in at number twenty on the list of the top two hundred products dispensed in the U.S. market in 2006, with 20,145,000 prescriptions.[2]

2. Digoxin (Trade Names: Digitek, Lanoxin, Lanoxicaps)

Digoxin is used for the treatment of congestive heart failure and to slow the ventricular rate in tachyarrhythmias (rapid, irregular heart-beats), such as atrial fibrillation, atrial flutter, and supraventricular tachycardia (cardiogenic shock). It essentially slows down the heart rate and lets it beat at the appropriate rate and rhythm.

This medication has many side effects, such as "heart block" (a delay in the transmission of the electrical signals that cause the heart to beat, leading to a much-too-slow heart rate), ventricular tachy-cardia or fibrillation, ST segment depression (changes on the EKG heart monitor), headache (3 percent), dizziness (5 percent), mental disturbances (4 percent), rash (2 percent), nausea, vomiting, diar-rhea (2–3 percent), and sometimes a general feeling of weakness. Digoxin is a medication that has a narrow therapeutic index, mean-ing that concentrations of this medication need to be maintained within a tight range. If the concentrations go above this range, which can happen easily because the range is so narrow, a patient might experience digoxin toxicity. Digoxin toxicity can manifest as nausea and vomiting in the earlier reaction stages that precede cardiotox-icity. A patient may also experience headache, visual disturbances ("halos" around lights), confusion, and disorientation.[3]

3. Warfarin (Trade Names: Coumadin, Jantoven)

Warfarin is used for prophylaxis (prevention) and treatment of thromboembolic (clotting) disorders and clotting complications caused by atrial fibrillation or cardiac valve replacement; it may also be used as an adjunct to reduce risk of systemic clot after a heart attack. It mainly works on vitamin K–dependent clotting factors. Warfarin inhibits these clotting factors, so the blood cannot form a clot as easily or quickly, thus preventing clots and the complications that accompany them.[4]

Bleeding is the main side effect of warfarin therapy. Other side effects include chest pain, low blood pressure, dizziness, fatigue, fe-ver, headache, rash, itching, joint or muscle pain, and a feeling of weakness. Bleeding is the most common adverse reaction associ-ated with warfarin and can appear as a variety of symptoms. People taking warfarin should watch for signs that include cuts that won't stop bleeding after applying pressure for fifteen to twenty minutes, bleeding from the gums or nose that won't stop, coughing up blood, stomach or abdominal pain, unusual swelling or pain, or unusual headache. Patients should become well informed about this medication before taking it. The following website offers more information: http://www.clevelandclinic.org/health/health-info/docs/2700/2790.asp?index=10001.

A black box warning states that warfarin may cause major or fatal bleeding. Risk factors for bleeding include high intensity anticoagulation (INR ≥4), age (≥65 years), variable INRs, history of GI (gastrointestinal) bleeding, high blood pressure, severe diabetes, trauma, and kidney problems. Skin necrosis/gangrene can occur but is very rare (≤0.1 percent). "Purple toe" syndrome due to microembolization has been rarely described with warfarin-type anticoagulants. (Microembolization involves small clots that decrease arterial blood flow.) This is not a common adverse reaction, and the purpose of mentioning it here is just to educate on the possibility of this rare reaction. Warfarin is also a pregnancy category X medication, meaning it should not be used during pregnancy. Patients should tell their doctors and/or dentists they are taking warfarin before having any kind of procedure performed, and they should not miss appointments to check their INRs.

 LET'S RECAP

Patient: Marty, age 70

1. Furosemide (Lasix) for water retention: 80 mg in morning, 40 mg in evening
2. Digoxin (Lanoxin) for heart rate control: 0.25 mg daily
3. Warfarin (Coumadin) for blood thinner; reduces clotting: 5 mg Monday, Tuesday, Thursday, Friday, Saturday; 7.5 mg Wednesday, Sunday

Lab-test results:

Digoxin: Within normal limits (normally 0.8–2.0 ng/mL)

INR (international normalized ratio): 9.1 (normally 2–3)

Potassium (K): 4.2 mEq/L (normally 3.5–5.2 mEq/L)

X-ray findings: Not applicable

SUMMARY REPORT

An initial evaluation of the situation suggests that Marty's heart condition and high cholesterol are not directly causing the symptoms and that the following information must be considered:

- Marty gets his digoxin serum (blood) concentrations checked at the ER, and he is within the normal therapeutic range (0.8–2.0 ng/mL, generally). We might have initially suspected that he is digoxin toxic because he has nausea and vomiting.

- His potassium levels are within the normal range also (4.2 mEq/L, with 3.5–5.2 mEq/L being normal). So, it most likely isn't the potassium causing the stomach upset and the feeling of unwellness.

- Bleeding is not a side effect of either furosemide or digoxin.

- Marty's INR is reported to be 9.1 (normally it should be between 2–3). The INR is a lab test that makes sure warfarin is working. It gives a doctor an idea of the balance between clotting and bleeding. Obviously, neither of these options should be out of the normal range. A doctor usually wants to check a patient's INR at least once a month, if not more often.

 SOLVE THE MYSTERY

Now we know that we can exclude digoxin and furosemide, because the lab tests came back normal and these medications do not have bleeding or bruising as a side effect. So guess what the culprit is?

 The Culprit: Warfarin

It should be noted that warfarin does have its risks along with its benefits. As noted previously, one of the major side effects of warfarin (Coumadin) is bleeding. Because Marty misses his last lab test after his doctor increases his dose, Marty has no idea his INR is so high. He should have made it to his lab appointment, and then he would have realized he has an increased INR that leads to his bleeding event. In Marty's case, he stops attending his lab appointments, and once his doctor increases his dose, Marty's INR jumps to 9.1, a very dangerous level. The main thing that starts Marty's bleeding incident is getting hit with the baseball. He develops a significant bleed, which likely leads to his loss of appetite and feeling of weakness (symptoms of anemia). Lab appointments are crucial in the proper management of a patient on warfarin and must not be missed.

THE SOLUTION

Warfarin acts on vitamin K–dependent clotting factors to prevent the blood from clotting; therefore, Marty is given vitamin K orally to reduce his INR. His INR and any signs of bleeding are monitored over the next forty-eight hours and every few days thereafter. Marty is instructed to discontinue his warfarin for a few days until the INR returns to the normal range (usually 2–3). Once his INR is back within the normal range, he is advised to resume a lower-dose regimen of warfarin (Coumadin).

WHAT ARE YOUR CHANCES?

It has been reported that the number of reported cases of warfarin-related bleeding has increased over the past few years. One study performed at the Harvard Medical School reported that up to 62 percent of the patients in the study received other medications that are known to increase/worsen the (bleeding) effects of warfarin.[5] Other sources suggest that the increase in the incidence of warfarin-related bleeding is also a reflection of the overall increase in the use of warfarin—that is, if more people are taking the drug, then more opportunities for an adverse event to happen arise.

One study found the incidence of first-time severe bleeding to be 2.3 per 100 patient-years.[6] Another study published in the *British Journal of General Practice* found that the incidence of fatal/hospitalized bleeding was 3.5 per 100 patient-years and incidence of referred bleeding was 2.6 per 100 patient-years, respectively.[7] To put things more simply, another article published in the *Annals of Internal Medicine* looked at thirty-three previously completed studies on warfarin use. It found that out of the 10,757 patients studied, 276 (2.5 percent) of them had a major bleeding event.[8] This calculates out to about a 1 in 39 chance of having a major bleeding event. Compare this with your chances of getting struck by lightning (in the United States). Your odds of being struck by lightning sometime in a year is 1 in 700,000.[9] (21,111,000 Rxs/12 Rxs per year for 1 patient = 1,759,250 patients × 2.5 percent = 43,981 major bleeds/ year.) In 2007 approximately 311 cases of INR elevations were reported to the FDA MedWatch system.[10] This figure does not include the multiple hemorrhages (bleeds) or other complications that were likely due to increased INRs.

Patient-year: A shorthand term used by epidemiologists to make comparisons; its value is determined by multiplying the number of individuals by the number of years the individuals' conditions were monitored. For example, one person followed for ten years or ten people followed for one year each equal ten patient-years.

HELPFUL ADVICE

Diet and other medications are a big factor in warfarin-related bleeding. Some studies have shown that the risk of developing bleeding depends on one's age, with people over age eighty being at a higher risk.[11] Let's just say that warfarin is a drug that needs to be taken very seriously. If you take it properly, get your INR checked regularly, eat consistently, and monitor the other medications you are taking, your chances of having a bleeding reaction probably aren't particularly high. However, if you are careless about taking medication, your chances of having a bleeding event may greatly increase. Marty should follow Rules #1, #6, and #7 to avoid this complication from reoccurring.

Be aware of and watch for the common signs of bleeding. Some common signs include blood in urine (dark red or brown urine), stool (black or red stools), or sputum (blood in your phlegm); bruises that are large and/or feel like they have a bump underneath; frequent nosebleeds; and cuts that won't stop bleeding (that is, they bleed for longer than fifteen minutes).

Vitamin K–dependent clotting factors (vitamin K is not to be confused with K+, which is the chemical abbreviation for potassium) are what warfarin acts on to prevent the blood from clotting. While taking warfarin, it is important to consistently eat foods with a high vitamin K content, such as spinach, collard greens, and kale (green, leafy vegetables). You are encouraged to and should eat these vegetables, as they provide many of the vitamins and nutrients you need in your diet. However, it is important to remember to be consistent with your diet. Don't just decide to immediately change to consuming a diet with high quantities of these vegetables, as this will decrease your INR dramatically. If you want to start such a diet, talk with your doctor first.

Always keep track of when you take your various medications. Some patients who take a lot of medicine find it difficult to remember when to take each medication; a pillbox or weekly pill planner is an easy way to organize your medications to ensure that you take the right ones at the right times. Most local pharmacies will even organize these boxes for you if you are unable to do it yourself. If you miss a dose, take it if it is within the same day, but do not double up on a dose the next day. Also, several drugs can interfere with warfarin and cause bleeding incidents. Avoid taking acetaminophen, aspirin, nonsteroidal anti-inflammatory drugs (NSAIDs), trimethoprim/sulfamethoxazole, erythromycin, amiodarone, propafenone, ketoconazole, fluconazole, itraconazole, and metronidazole. Some drugs can increase bleeds and should be avoided if you are elderly, such as quinolones (ciprofloxacin, levofloxacin), omeprazole, clarithromycin, and azithromycin. If you are prescribed any of these, you should be alerted to how they interact with warfarin.[12]

Tips for People Taking Warfarin

Here are some tips to help prevent falls in the home: Remove loose rugs and electrical cords that could lead to tripping, slipping, or falling; ensure that all areas of the house include adequate lighting; and avoid walking on ice, polished floors, wet floors, or in unfamiliar areas outside of your house.

It is also a good idea to wear medical identification, such as a bracelet or necklace, to notify health-care providers and others that you are taking warfarin. Most local pharmacies have the ability to order these for you, and they can be mailed right to your home within a few days.

In addition, it is important not only to watch what you eat but also what you drink. Grapefruit juice, cranberry juice, and alcoholic beverages are three of the main drinks to limit or to avoid when taking certain medications. They can alter the metabolism of your medications and should be avoided with warfarin. Also, warfarin comes in multiple strengths. One easy way to make sure you are getting the right strength is to look at the tablet color. Each strength of warfarin is a distinct color and should always be that same color. For example, Coumadin 5 mg is a peach color, while Coumadin 6 mg is teal or blue-green. Checking the color is an easy way to make sure your doctor and pharmacy refilled your prescription correctly. The color is consistent across the generic brands, but the pills may not be identical; for example, they may differ in shape with one being oval and another square.

 VIOLATION OF RULE #1: Learn from Others—What Is Happening in the ER?

Like digoxin, warfarin is one of the leading causes of visits to the ER due to drug reactions. Had Marty been more careful and known how dangerous this medication was, he may have been more inclined to be cautious while taking warfarin. As a patient you should report any signs and symptoms of bleeding (nosebleeds; easy bruising; blood in your urine, stool, or sputum; and fatigue) to your doctor.

VIOLATION OF RULE #6: Know Your Lab-Test Schedule

Along the same lines, Marty should have realized how dangerous warfarin is and followed his lab-test schedule and been aware of his monitoring parameters. Marty and any patient taking warfarin should have their INRs checked at least monthly.

 VIOLATION OF RULE #7: Know Your Medication's Monitoring Parameters

For most patients, the INR should be between 2 and 3 (up to 3.5 in some patients). This is usually your doctor's target range to make sure you aren't at risk for clots (INR less than 2) or at risk for bleeding (INR above 3). Neither one is a good option, so again, have your INR checked every month. Here are three good questions to ask yourself after you have your INR checked:

1. What was my result (keep a log of your INR values)?
2. Do I need to change my warfarin dose based on this result?
3. When should I have my next blood draw?[13]

CONDITION

Medication-Induced Upper-GI Bleeding

The following case shows us that some medications can cause upper-GI bleeding. Upper-GI bleeding is bleeding from the upper gastrointestinal tract, including the esophagus, stomach, and duodenum (the first section of the small intestine).

 THE PATIENT

Betty is a fifty-seven-year-old woman with a history of heart problems. She has always had high blood pressure and within the past few years has learned she also has high cholesterol. On top of all that, she is also a type 2 diabetic. A couple of years ago, Betty had a heart attack. She has also undergone coronary bypass surgery. She used to smoke when she was younger but stopped several years ago. Her doctor has advised her to take an aspirin every day to help her heart and to help prevent another heart attack.

THE SYMPTOMS

Lately, Betty has been feeling more tired than usual, and some days she can hardly get up and go. She has also noticed that she is becoming increasingly short of breath. Today her symptoms seem to be getting worse. She is starting to have abdominal pain and cramping, feels weak, and is also experiencing dizziness. She *really* starts to worry when she vomits and it looks like coffee grounds. Betty realizes she has had some trouble in the past and knows that she is no spring chicken, but she still thinks these symptoms are not normal for a fairly active fifty-seven-year-old woman. It is not as though she's ninety years old (although regardless of age, these symptoms should be checked). What could be going on with Betty?

THE SUSPECTS

The likely suspects are the following drugs.

1. Aspirin (Trade Names: Bayer, Ecotrin, Ascriptin, Bufferin, Easprin, St. Joseph Adult Aspirin)

Aspirin treats pain and fever and also reduces the risk of death in heart attack and strokes by decreasing platelet clotting. It can cause nausea, vomiting, and dizziness. The chemical structure name is acetylsalicylic acid (ASA). Aspirin is an NSAID, and taking it with other NSAIDs may decrease platelet effect, which means that less blood clotting and a higher chance of bleeding could result. Aspirin is also in the subclass of salicylates that can cause Reye's syndrome in children. For more information on Reye's syndrome, visit http://cks.library.nhs.uk/patient_information_leaflet/reyes_syndrome.[14]

2. Glyburide (Trade Names: Diaßeta, Glynase, PresTab, Micronase)

Glyburide is used for the oral management of type 2 diabetes mellitus to stimulate insulin release. Some of the reported reactions include headache, dizziness, rash, nausea/vomiting, hypoglycemia (blood sugar that is too low), anemia, and heartburn. Hypoglycemia can occur with glyburide. With regular high doses of aspirin, the two drugs can interact to enhance glyburide's hypoglycemic effect.[15]

3. Atorvastatin (Trade Name: Lipitor)

Atorvastatin is used for the treatment of high cholesterol and/or prevention of (atherosclerotic) heart disease. It reduces total cholesterol and LDL ("bad") cholesterol. Headache (3–17 percent) is the most common side effect of atorvastatin. Other reactions that may occur in 2 to 10 percent of patients include chest pain, edema (fluid retention), dizziness, rash, diarrhea or constipation, increased liver functions, and muscle pain and/or cramping. A few rare but serious side effects are rhabdomyolysis (breakdown of muscle that presents as random and unexplained muscle pain), Stevens-Johnson syndrome (burnlike rash), and Achilles tendon rupture. Atorvastatin should not be used during pregnancy.[16]

LET'S RECAP

Patient: Betty, age 57
1. Aspirin for preventing blood clots. 325 mg daily
2. Glyburide (many) for diabetes: 2.5 mg daily
3. Atorvastatin (Lipitor) for high cholesterol: 20 mg at bedtime
Lab-test results: All within normal limits
X-ray findings: Not applicable

SUMMARY REPORT

An initial evaluation suggests that Betty's heart condition is not causing these symptoms. The following information must be considered:

- Betty checks her blood sugar, and it is 148 (normal range 90–130), which is actually a pretty good reading for Betty.

Hint: Many poorly controlled diabetics may have readings in the 200s or even the 300 to 400 range (see the case of Kristi Jo in Chapter 3, "Are Your Meds Causing Kidney, Calcium, Liver, Pancreas, or Diabetic Complications?").

- Betty takes what is considered a "low dose" of aspirin each day, one 325 mg tablet. Hint: Most sources consider anything from 75 to 325 mg of aspirin daily to be a low dose.[17]

- Betty does not have any particular muscle pain and has been taking the same dose of atorvastatin (Lipitor) for a few years now, which has never made her sick before.

- The coffee-grounds appearance of Betty's vomit indicates that she has an upper GI (gastrointestinal/stomach) bleed.

SOLVE THE MYSTERY

We can pretty much rule out all her medications, except aspirin, as possible culprits. We know that she has a GI bleed. Which of these medications is the most likely to cause her to have a stomach ulcer or bleed?

The Culprit: Aspirin

Aspirin has caused Betty to develop a small GI bleed, and this is what is making her feel so bad. The GI tract includes the esophagus, stomach, small intestine, large intestine (colon), rectum, and anus. Bleeding can occur from any one of these areas. Bleeding can even occur without a person's noticing it (also known as occult bleeding). Such medications as aspirin and NSAIDs can be hard on the stomach if taken in high doses and/or if taken on an empty stomach. Come to find out, Betty always takes her aspirin first thing in the morning, about an hour before she has breakfast.

THE SOLUTION

Betty spends a couple of days in the hospital to make sure the bleeding stops and that her other blood tests are normal. She is prescribed a medication (proton pump inhibitor [PPI]) to help prevent stomach ulceration/upset by reducing the acid in the stomach. Betty's doctor has also decided to drop her aspirin dose down to that of a baby aspirin, or an 81 mg chewable aspirin a day, and has instructed her to be sure to take the aspirin with food, and not on an empty stomach. Even though she did suffer this stomach bleed, the doctor still feels that the aspirin's heart benefits outweigh the risk of her developing another GI bleed.

WHAT ARE YOUR CHANCES?

A slight controversy exists regarding the actual rate or incidence of aspirin-induced GI bleed. One journal reported that the annualized rate of upper GI bleed was 1.2 events per 100 patient-years.[18] This journal article also noted that low-dose aspirin carries a small but significant risk for upper GI bleed and that the lowest dose of aspirin is probably safest.

Another study that was conducted in Denmark found the rate of hospitalization for upper GI bleeding in its population (about twenty-seven thousand patients) who were using aspirin but no other anticoagulants was about 0.06 percent per year.[19]

Aspirin is one of the most frequent causes of ulceration, and 10 to 15 percent of patients taking aspirin for rheumatoid arthritis will have an ulcer after one month. The risk of an ulcer increases with doses from 2.5 percent for doses less than 100 mg to 15 percent for higher doses used to treat rheumatoid arthritis. The stomach is the most common site of these ulcers.[20]

Risk factors of an ulceration due to aspirin use include a prior ulceration or GI complication, prolonged use, being elderly, using an anticoagulation agent (warfarin) or corticosteroid, and using aspirin and NSAIDs together.[21] According to the FDA's MedWatch reporting system, aspirin was responsible for approximately ninety-eight GI bleeds in 2007.[22] This accounts for multiple GI hemorrhages (bleeds) that were reported to the FDA. The data were pooled as multiple variations of GI bleeds and reported as intestinal, gastric, and duodenal.

HELPFUL ADVICE

A patient taking a low-dose aspirin, usually 81 mg, should be aware of the signs of bleeding; however, the average patient has a very low risk of developing a GI bleed. When combined with other medications that could increase bleeding, more caution should be exercised. Always ask a physician or pharmacist prior to beginning any medication that carries this risk. Many sources show a decreased risk of having a bleed with aspirin use when patients used medications known as PPIs (proton pump inhibitors, such as omeprazole 20 mg daily). If you are on aspirin, I recommend asking your doctor whether starting a PPI is appropriate for you. Betty should have read Rule #10.[23]

You may be able to help prevent GI bleed by using low(er)-dose aspirin (81 mg). Ulcers are not reduced by using enteric-coated aspirin.[24] Enteric coating means that the drug has a delayed-release safety coating. As mentioned earlier, you should also try to avoid taking aspirin on an empty stomach. PPIs may help decrease the risk of a GI bleed.

Be aware of the signs and symptoms of bleeding. If the bleeding is occurring in the rectum or lower colon, bright red blood will coat or mix with the stool. When bleeding is happening in the esophagus, stomach, or small intestine, the stool may look black or tarry.[25] If you are losing blood, you may also become anemic. Anemia (reduced red blood cells) may make you feel weak, dizzy, faint, or short of breath, and it can cause abdominal pain or diarrhea. If untreated, shock may also occur. Signs of shock may include rapid pulse, decreased blood pressure, not making urine, and pale skin color.

VIOLATION OF RULE #10: Understand That Over-the-Counter Medicines, Herbals, and Alcohol Are All Drugs

Although aspirin may seem like a benign medication, it is not. Aspirin has the ability to send you or a loved one to the hospital with a serious GI bleed. In Betty's case, she is taking what is considered a low dose of aspirin to prevent heart disease, and she winds up in the emergency room with a serious bleed. Be careful when taking aspirin, and follow these suggestions: First, know what to look for when it comes to detecting a GI bleed. If you notice any unusual stomach pains or cramps, unusual heartburn or what seems to be acid reflux, vomit that resembles coffee grounds, and dark "tarry" or bright red stools, contact your doctor. Second, talk with your doctor about starting a PPI (omeprazole, lansoprazole, or pantoprazole). This class of medications can reduce the risk of having a GI bleed related to aspirin. Take aspirin with meals and a full glass of water.

CONDITION

Medication-Induced Gastrointestinal Ulceration

The following case shows us that some medications can cause gastrointestinal ulceration, an ulcer that can cause bleeding anywhere throughout the gastrointestinal (GI tract)—from the mouth to the anus.

THE PATIENT

Beverly is a fifty-five-year-old woman who considers herself to be fairly healthy. Since her fiftieth birthday, Beverly has become much more active and involved with her overall health care. She has been trying to watch her diet and exercise more often. She goes for walks every day. Beverly has had back problems in the past, and even though her pain is much improved since her back surgery, she still has some pain on a day-to-day basis. She takes an over-the-counter (OTC) NSAID for the pain. Her blood pressure has also been high in the past, for which she takes a combination blood pressure medication called Vaseretic. She also has early signs of osteoporosis (weakening of the bone). She and her doctor decide to try Fosamax (alendronate) to help prevent bone loss after she watches a commercial promoting this medication.

THE SYMPTOMS

Beverly has noticed some weight loss over the past month or two. Actually, she has lost more than ten pounds in the past few weeks. At first, Beverly is really excited by this weight loss, because she thinks her dieting and exercising efforts are finally kicking in. She has also noticed that she gets significant heartburn after meals, and over the last week or so she has felt nauseated and has had intermittent vomiting. She has also become increasingly weak and dizzy. Now she just feels really bloated, and her belly is distended. Her stomach is hurting her severely, so she decides to have her husband take her to the ER to find out what is going on.

THE SUSPECTS

The likely suspects are the following drugs.

1. Enalapril, Hydrochlorothiazide (Trade Name: Vaseretic)

Vaseretic is used for the treatment of high blood pressure and/or edema associated with congestive heart failure. Side effects include hypotension (1–7 percent), chest pain (2 percent), fainting (0.5–2 percent), headache (2–5 percent), dizziness (4–8 percent), fatigue (2–3 percent), abnormal taste, abdominal pain, vomiting, nausea, diarrhea or constipation, cough, orthostatic hypotension (blood pressure drops too low upon standing), photosensitivity, hypokalemia (low potassium), and loss of appetite and/or pain in the epigastric region (that is, the upper-middle area of the abdomen). Angioedema (swelling beneath the skin) is a rare but serious side effect that may occur when taking angiotensin-converting enzyme (ACE) inhibitors, such as Vaseretic (enalapril and hydrochlorothiazide). Vaseretic carries a black box warning that says to avoid use during pregnancy. ACE inhibitors can cause injury and death to a developing fetus when used in the second and third trimesters. Discontinue ACE inhibitors as soon as pregnancy is detected.[26]

2. Alendronate (Trade Name: Fosamax)

Alendronate is used for the treatment and/or prevention for osteoporosis in men and women. It helps prevent breakdown of bones. Side effects associated with this medication include transient increase in calcium (18 percent), transient decrease in phosphorous (10 percent), headache (2–3 percent), abdominal pain (1–7 percent), acid reflux (1–4 percent), upset stomach (1–4 percent), nausea (1–4 percent), flatulence (up to 4 percent), diarrhea (1–3 percent), gastroesophageal reflux disease (1–3 percent), constipation (up to 3 percent), esophageal ulcer (up to 2 percent), abdominal distension (up to 1 percent), gastritis (up to 1 percent), vomiting (up to 1 percent), trouble swallowing (up to 1 percent), gastric ulcer (1 percent), and muscle pain (up to 6 percent).[27]

Alendronate must be taken with plain water (tablets, 6–8 oz. water; oral solution, follow with 2 oz. water) first thing in the morning and approximately thirty minutes before the first food, beverage other than water (this medication should not be taken with mineral water or with other beverages), or other medication of the day. After taking alendronate, patients should not lie down and must remain in the upright position (standing if possible) for at least thirty minutes and until after the first food of the day (to reduce esophageal irritation). Patients should receive supplemental calcium and vitamin D if dietary intake is inadequate.[28]

3. Naproxen (Trade Names: Aleve, Naprosyn)

Naproxen reduces mild-to-moderate pain and may be used for the management of ankylosing spondylitis, osteoarthritis, or rheumatoid disorders. It also may be used to treat pain caused by gout, tendonitis, bursitis, dysmenorrhea, or fever. It works by inhibiting cyclooxygenase (COX) and prostaglandin synthesis, which are both responsible for/cause pain and inflammation. Naproxen can cause abdominal pain, constipation, nausea, heartburn, headache, edema, and dizziness or drowsiness (all 3–9 percent). It may also cause GI ulceration and bleeding and kidney problems. Naproxen belongs to a class of drugs called NSAIDs.[29]

LET'S RECAP

Patient: Beverly, age 55

1. Enalapril and hydrochlorothiazide (Vaseretic) for high blood pressure: one (10-25*) tablet daily
2. Alendronate (Fosamax) for Osteoporosis: 70 mg tab weekly
3. Naproxen (Aleve, Anaprox, Naproxsyn) for inflammation/pain: 1–2 times daily, as needed for back pain

Lab-test results: All within normal limits

X-ray findings: Not applicable

---

* 10-25 is the appropriate way to express the dosage for this combination drug. It reflects the concentrations of both enalapril and hydrochlorathiazide in the medication.

SUMMARY REPORT

An initial evaluation of the situation suggests that Beverly's symptoms are not due to any previously known disease. The following information must be considered:

- Beverly is taking Naproxen for her back pain, but her doctor doesn't know how much she takes.

- Beverly likes to drink orange juice first thing in the morning. After she drinks her glass of orange juice, she likes to relax and recline in the chair. This is not how alendronate (Fosamax) is supposed to be taken.

- Beverly was working out in the yard the other day and has since noticed an increase in the pain in her back. She knows she shouldn't have been pulling those weeds. She has been taking two naproxen (Aleve) tablets a day, the recommended dose.

- When Beverly gets to the hospital, the doctors do a procedure called an endoscopy and discover that she has a couple of small ulcerations. One of the ulcerations is in her lower esophagus, and the other one is in the stomach.

- Fosamax has a warning in its package insert against the use of this alendronate with NSAIDs. In clinical trials, the use of both increased the risk for GI bleeds.

The Culprit: Alendronate (Fosamax)

As with other bisphosphonates (such as Boniva and Actonel), these drugs can cause esophageal ulceration when not taken as instructed. Beverly does not take her alendronate with plain water; she takes it with orange juice. Orange juice is acidic and may increase stomach irritation. She also likes to recline in the chair after taking her medication. It is very important to remain either standing or sitting in the upright position for at least thirty minutes after taking this medication. If possible, it is even better to remain in this upright position for an hour after taking the medication. It is also important to take alendronate on an empty stomach.[30]

The Accomplice: Naproxen

Beverly is also taking a naproxen (Aleve) tablet twice a day. Each tablet contains 220 mg of naproxen. The maximum recommended dose per day of naproxen is 600 mg. Beverly is taking less than the recommended amount; however, naproxen can still cause GI bleeds, especially when taken in high doses.

The combination of naproxen and alendronate increases the risk for the development of gastric ulcers. Either of these medications alone carries a high risk for developing GI ulceration, but when used in combination, it has been shown to more than triple the risk of stomach ulcers.[31]

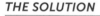 *THE SOLUTION*

Beverly is started on intravenous pantoprazole (Protonix) while in the hospital, and her bleeding is monitored. She remains hospitalized for a couple of days. When the doctor is sure she isn't bleeding anymore, and when her lab-test results are all back to normal, she is allowed to go home. The physician sends her home with a prescription for a PPI (Prevacid) as well. She is instructed to avoid taking NSAIDs (ibuprofen, naproxen, and aspirin are the most commonly used). The doctor increases the dose of her other pain medication. Acetaminophen, which is not an NSAID, can achieve similar benefits of pain relief with minimal, if any, impact on the stomach lining.[32] Bev is also instructed on the proper use of alendronate (Fosamax). It has strict instructions on how to take it for a reason—follow them!

WHAT ARE YOUR CHANCES?

As mentioned before, your chances for developing a GI bleed from certain medications may be fairly high. NSAIDs and bisphosphonates especially carry a high risk. Because many NSAIDs are available over the counter (such as Aleve, Advil, Motrin, and aspirin), this is a big concern.

It has been noted that more than ninety-five million people in the United States experience some kind of digestive problem each year, more than ten million people are hospitalized annually, and total health-care costs exceed $40 billion each year.[33] NSAIDs are reported to be the second major cause for ulcers or irritation to the stomach.

An estimated 1 to 3 percent of patients taking NSAIDs (naproxen, ibuprofen) will develop a GI bleed.[34] A meta-analysis of recent trials found the absolute rate increase of having a GI bleed due to low-dose aspirin as compared with a placebo was about 0.12 percent per year.[35] Consider the statistics of the number of people (approximately 303,264,200)[36] in the United States versus the number of people who are hospitalized each year for GI problems (10,000,000).[37] A little more than 3 percent of people in the United States are hospitalized for GI problems.

It is fair to say that when taken at or below the OTC recommended dosages, NSAIDs are safe and effective, and your chances of developing a GI bleed are low. However, when you ingest more than the recommended dose, take NSAIDs for more than ten days, or add a medication, such as alendronate (Fosamax), your risk goes up.

Some risk factors for NSAID-related GI adverse effects include being over age sixty, having a history of peptic ulcer disease, concurrently using corticosteroids, concurrently using anticoagulation medication, and taking high doses of NSAIDs.[38] The incidence of gastroduodenal ulcer from various NSAID use after twelve weeks of therapy is 35 percent for naproxen, 23 to 29 percent for ibuprofen, 10 percent for diclofenac, 7 percent for celecoxib, and 4 to 7 percent for placebo.[39]

An incidence of patients taking both NSAIDs and alendronate (Fosamax) could not be located. However, according to the FDA's MedWatch reporting system, fifty-seven cases of GI ulceration, GI bleed, and other symptoms of GI bleeds due to naproxen were reported in 2007. A search of the MedWatch system turned up fifty-seven cases of gastric (stomach) ulcers, esophageal bleed, and esophageal ulceration due to Fosamax in 2007. Given the incidence of GI bleeds with each of the two medications, combining them can only increase the risk of a GI bleed.[40]

HELPFUL ADVICE

Patients taking both of these medications should be very cautious and aware of bleeding complications. Other medications should be tried prior to starting NSAIDs in combination with bisphosphonates. Many people are admitted to the hospital every year with some sort of GI bleed. Taking medications that increase this risk is dangerous, but the benefits of therapy should be weighed prior to initiating treatment. In the future, Beverly should abide by Rules #7 and #10 to prevent this complication from recurring.

Maybe one of the most important things you can do while taking NSAIDs is to always try to take them with food or milk. This will help protect the stomach and decrease the risk of ulcers.

Once again, be aware of the signs and symptoms associated with GI bleeding. When the doctor questions Beverly about any signs of blood in her stool, she first replies no. Then, when the doctor asks her whether she has recently noticed any black or tarry stools, she replies yes. Thus, if Beverly had known that black or tarry stools are a sign of bleeding, she may have gotten to the hospital sooner. Remember to also look for signs of dark clots or coffee grounds–like material if vomiting, and look for bright red blood mixed in or with the stool. Any pain, particularly pain behind the breastbone, should also be reported.

When it comes to taking alendronate (Fosamax), follow the directions. The package directions are specific for a reason: The drug can be dangerous if not taken properly. Take alendronate first thing in the morning with at least 6 to 8 ounces of water (not juice, not coffee, not even mineral water). Take alendronate on an empty stomach (not with breakfast). Swallow the tablet whole (do not crush or chew the tablet). Do not lie back down or even recline your chair if you must sit for at least thirty minutes. Yes, this means standing for thirty minutes. If you can't stand for that long, sit in an upright position; do not use a recliner. I recommend that every three months you get your basic lab tests, including checking levels of blood urea nitrogen (BUN) and serum creatinine (SCr), rechecked. Alendronate may not be the best option for you if you have esophageal abnormalities, if you have low calcium levels in your blood, if you can't stand or sit upright for thirty minutes, and if you are at risk for aspiration (in which foreign substances or solids/liquids that belong in the stomach are breathed into the lungs instead).[41]

 VIOLATION OF RULE #5: Take Your Medication as Your Doctor Prescribed

Beverly is not careful about following the directions and taking her medication exactly as prescribed. She fails to talk with her doctor about starting naproxen (Aleve) for back pain. Had she asked her pharmacist or physician about taking naproxen with alendronate (Fosamax), she would have been warned about the possible risks associated with using both medications at the same time. She also does not know what to look for if she is having a GI (gastrointestinal) bleed. Take alendronate exactly as prescribed, and follow the package directions. Alendronate is a great drug that helps your bones and prevents osteoporosis, but it has some serious side effects that you should be aware of.

VIOLATION OF RULE #10: Understand That Over-the-Counter Medicines, Herbals, and Alcohol Are All Drugs

As mentioned, Beverly and everyone else who is taking an NSAID or alendronate should report any stomach pain/cramps; frequent heartburn; unusual vomit that resembles coffee grounds; dark, tarry, or bright red stools; and any pain that seems to be located behind your sternum (breastbone). Beverly did not show all of these symptoms, but they can all be signs of serious GI complications from your medications. Also, when taking Fosamax, be aware of a rare but serious side effect that causes pain in the jaw. Inform your dentist that you take alendronate. If you notice unusual jaw pain, contact your doctor.

 VIOLATION OF RULE #16: Ads Don't Warn of Incidence of Adverse Events—Don't Believe Them

Have you ever noticed Advil commercials? One features a lovely, blond actress suffering from a cold, and she is in her house blowing her nose and looking miserable. The next thing you know, she is swimming laps in the pool, just like that. Everything looks fine and dandy, but again no one even mentions any risks or incidence of adverse events. The only warning in the entire commercial is a small phrase at the bottom of the screen put up for about a second that reads, "Make sure this drug is right for you. Read and follow the label." This is why this book points out the risk of bleeding from NSAIDs and warns you to be aware of such complications in order to prevent them.

CHAPTER 6

Are Your Meds Causing Strange and Unusual Symptoms?

It is important to report to your doctor any unusual symptoms you may have after taking a medication, including any changes in bowel habits, rashes, or dizziness.

CONDITION

Medication-Induced Intestinal Blockage

The following case shows us that some medications can make your intestines stop working, resulting in a blockage that prevents food from passing through the intestines.

THE PATIENT

Stella is a seventy-two-year-old retired schoolteacher. When able to participate, she is an active member of the community. Stella currently lives alone. Her husband passed away several years ago from colon-cancer complications. Stella has a laundry list of medical conditions that have slowed her down over the past years. Despite being a mentor to young students, Stella lets her diabetes care and control slip. As a result of the nonadherence to her diabetic treatment, she has many complications, such as decreased kidney function and stomach problems. She has had a stroke and has hypertension. Also, she suffers from severe nerve pain from the diabetes. Her doctor has placed her on a strong pain medication (oxycodone) to help her obtain some relief.

THE SYMPTOMS

Stella is awakened by a terrible pain in her stomach. She also feels like she could throw up at anytime. She calls a friend to take her to the hospital. Once at the hospital, Stella tells the doctor that she hasn't had a bowel movement for four days even though she has been taking a laxative. Stella is distraught by the thought of having another illness and having to take more medication. After running a few tests, the doctor determines that Stella's stomach problem is not directly caused by her medical conditions, so to solve the case he focuses on her medications.

THE SUSPECTS

The likely suspects are the following drugs.

1. Metoclopramide (Trade Name: Reglan)

Metoclopramide treats symptoms of diabetic gastric stasis (digestive tract not working properly) and gastrointestinal reflux. It may cause drowsiness (10–70 percent), fatigue (approximately 10 percent), muscle spasms and dyskinesias (uncontrolled movements), and restlessness (approximately 10 percent). Metoclopramide is considered a prokinetic, which means by its molecular actions it increases gastric motility and stimulates gastric emptying.[1]

2. Oxycodone (Trade Name: OxyContin or OxyIR)

Oxycodone is used for the management of moderate to severe pain and can cause somnolence (sleepiness; 24 percent), dizziness (14 percent), constipation (26 percent), and nausea (14 percent). This drug carries a black box warning that health professionals should be aware of its potential for abuse, misuse, and diversion. Because of this, oxycodone is considered a controlled substance. Oxycodone is a controlled-release formulation that should be taken regularly and not merely as needed, because the drug is released over twelve hours and is not as effective for acute problems. This formulation should also never be crushed or chewed.

3. Docusate (Trade Name: Colace)[2]

Docusate is a stool softener and can cause stomach cramping and diarrhea in 1 to 10 percent of patients. A stool softener does not stimulate a bowel movement, but it makes it easier for a bowel movement to move out of the lower digestive tract. Docusate is an over-the-counter (OTC) medication that is commonly used by elderly patients. Constipation is one of the most common gastrointestinal complaints in the United States. More than 4 million Americans have frequent constipation, accounting for 2.5 million physician visits a year.[2] Those reporting constipation most often are women and adults ages sixty-five or older. Pregnant women may have constipation, and it is a common problem following childbirth or surgery.[3] Self-treatment of constipation with OTC laxatives is by far the most common remedy. Approximately $725 million is spent on laxative products each year in the United States.[4]

LET'S RECAP

Patient: Stella, age 72
1. Metoclopramide (Reglan) for diabetic gastroparesis: 5 mg 4 times a day
2. Oxycodone (OxyContin) for pain control: 80 mg 2 times a day
3. Docusate (Colace) for constipation: 100 mg 4 times a day
Lab-test results: All within normal limits
X-ray findings: X ray shows small bowel obstruction with stool impaction

SUMMARY REPORT

The problem is not caused directly by one of Stella's medical conditions. The following information must be considered:

- The doses of all her medications are within normal limits.
- Docusate and metoclopramide are used to help Stella's stomach problems.
- An X ray shows an impaction in the bowel.

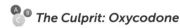

The Culprit: Oxycodone

Constipation is a common side effect of oxycodone. It has been reported in about 26 percent of patients.[5] OxyContin (oxycodone) had its biggest year in 2000, with 5.8 million prescriptions sold.[6] This number has decreased somewhat (but not significantly) due to its widespread abuse. The constipation is a result of the opiate-type medication's directly slowing down the digestive tract. The slowing of the tract leads to longer transit time for stool moving through the large intestine, so more water is absorbed from the stool. Therefore, hardened stool forms in the digestive tract.[7] It is also possible that Stella's gastrointestinal system may have already been impaired in terms of contracting to move food through the digestive process (peristalsis). This slowing may be due to gastroparesis, a condition in which the stomach takes too long to empty its food contents into the small intestine. Gastroparesis is a common adverse consequence of diabetes, but age is also a factor that contributes to a slower gastrointestinal tract action. Because of this decrease in digestive tract's ability to move, Stella takes metoclopramide and docusate. The addition of the very constipating oxycodone precipitated the hardened stool obstruction.

THE SOLUTION

Stella is given intravenous fluids to keep her hydrated and to maintain electrolytes. She is restricted from eating and drinking to allow her stomach and intestine to rest. She is given some stimulating laxatives that are considered powerful. Stella may have to have surgery to correct the blockage, but a surgeon will make that determination based on what effects the blockage is having on her intestines. Stella's physician also needs to determine whether she is benefiting enough from the oxycodone to keep her on it.

WHAT ARE YOUR CHANCES?

One review of literature showed that 12 to 19 percent of Americans are affected with constipation. One of the major causes of constipation is pain medications (opioids/narcotics). In one study, 95 percent of patients who were interviewed by nurses in an oncology unit reported constipation as a side effect of their pain medications. A meta-analysis reviewing eleven studies of patients with chronic, noncancer pain revealed that 41 percent of patients experienced constipation (the most common side effect). These patients were on oral potent opioids (morphine, methadone, hydromorphone, or fentanyl).[8] No data exist that give the exact percentage of patients who will experience a bowel obstruction from the constipation caused by opiate (oxycodone) medications. One manufacturer of oxycodone that was contacted acknowledged that constipation-induced bowel obstructions were a known event but was not able to provide figures for the incidence. One source stated that less than 5 percent of small bowel obstructions are due to miscellaneous causes, and opiate-induced fecal impaction was in this category.

Fecal impaction secondary to constipation occurs more commonly in children and older adults.[9] Other sources place the number of patients experiencing constipation from opiates at up to 90 percent.[10] The incidence of drug-induced constipation in opioids varies with differing agents. Some examples of the incidence of constipations include codeine at 10 to 21 percent, fentanyl at 3.7 to 27 percent, morphine at 5.1 to 57 percent, and oxycodone at 6.1 to 23 percent.[11]

A search of FDA's MedWatch system turned up a reported thirty-two cases of constipation for 2007.[12] However, most patients taking opioids for chronic pain have difficulty with constipation. Constipation is a real problem for many patients, so talk with your doctor or pharmacist if you experience this reaction.

HELPFUL ADVICE

Constipation is a common issue with opioid drugs. Fortunately, the vast majority of cases do not result in hospitalization. If you are on chronic opioid therapy, statistics say you will experience constipation. The best way to stay out of the hospital is to avoid the problem by taking preventative laxative therapy with a stimulant. Using lower doses of the opioid medication will not prevent constipation, because the dosage that produces constipation is four times smaller than the analgesic (pain-relieving) dose.[13] Also, following Rule #4 in this case may have led to a decreased chance of hospitalization.

Stella is also on a high dose of oxycodone. She is not on any other opioid medications and therefore is not tolerant to its effects. She should have been on a lower dose, such as 10 mg every twelve hours. This lower dose would not have prevented constipation, but the high dose of oxycodone could have led to other serious adverse events, such as respiratory depression. Rule #15 should also have been followed.

Make sure all health-care professionals are aware of what you take and of the diseases you have. By practicing this vigilance, your care will be more efficient. In Stella's case, she is diabetic, and her physician should have realized that significant constipation is a serious consequence of placing her on oxycodone. Her physician must weigh the benefits of reduced pain with the risks of sedation and constipation prevalent with oxycodone therapy.

While on opiates or other constipating drugs, be aware of your bowel habits. Remember, constipation is defined as having fewer than three bowel movements a week. A person does not have to go every day, but if you are on a pain medication and have not had a bowel movement for two days, consult your physician. Monitor for abnormal abdominal pain and nausea and vomiting, as these are common signs of constipation.

Some relief measures that you may take while on constipating medications are to increase your fluid intake and to increase your physical activity as much as possible. I recommend taking any of the following laxatives while on chronic opioid treatment: stool softeners (docusate [Colace], Doc-Q-Lace, Kristalose, Enulose, Milk of Magnesia, Miralax), stimulants (bisacodyl, senna), or a combination of the above (docusate/senna). When stimulant laxatives are used correctly, they do not cause problems and are not harmful to the colon. If you do not respond to stool softeners, stimulant laxatives may be used chronically, but combination laxatives provide the best therapy.[14]

VIOLATION OF RULE #4: Be Aware That Elderly Patients Are Different from Younger People

It is well known that many elderly patients suffer from constipation without confounding factors, such as Stella's. She is a diabetic who is already on two medications to prevent constipation and to help with her digestive tract. She should have been wary when her physician suggested that she try oxycodone. Had she been more inquisitive, she, along with her physician, may have realized that oxycodone may not have been the most appropriate pain medication to try. Fiber laxatives/bulk producers (Metamucil, Citrucel, FiberCon, Benefiber, and Maltsupex) are prime examples of laxatives that can *worsen* the constipation seen with opioids by inhibiting movement of the GI tract. Instead, try a stimulant laxative, such as senna or bisacodyl, to relieve your symptoms. Be aware of the symptoms of constipation, such as abdominal pain, cramping, nausea and vomiting. Remember, if you have not had a bowel movement in two to three days, talk to your physician or pharmacist about options to remedy the situation.

VIOLATION OF RULE #15: Remember That Elderly Individuals Should Be on Lower Doses

Stella's dosage of oxycodone is also too high. Even though following Rule #15 may not have prevented constipation, it may have prevented other side effects from occurring. Stella is elderly, and this dose is too high for her age. This could have resulted in a fall or even worse complications. Make sure that you are on the correct dose for your age.

███████ **CONDITION** ███████

Medication-Induced Lactic Acidosis

The following case shows us that some medications can cause lactic acidosis. Lactic acidosis is a condition in which there is too much acid in the body due to a buildup of lactic acid.

THE PATIENT

James is a fifty-five-year-old man with high blood pressure, chronic obstructive pulmonary disease (COPD), heartburn, and a recent diagnosis of type 2 diabetes. He started smoking when he was fifteen years old but gave up the butts ten years ago. However, when he quit smoking, he started drinking more, and now he has a beer with lunch and dinner and a whiskey sour before bed every night.

THE SYMPTOMS

When James wakes up this morning, he just can't get moving. He tells his wife, Shirley, that it feels like his heart is beating too slowly, that he is so tired, and that all his muscles hurt very badly. He feels as though he just ran a marathon. Shirley already knows something is wrong, because never in their twenty-seven years of marriage has James hogged the bedcovers unless he is sick. Shirley calls their doctor, Dr. Louie, after James doesn't get up for two more hours. Dr. Louie says, "You know, Shirley, why don't I meet you and James at the hospital, just to check out his heart to be safe?"

THE SUSPECTS

The likely suspects are the following drugs.

1. Metformin (Trade Name: Glucophage)

Metformin is the mainstay in oral treatment of type 2 adult diabetes. It works by decreasing glucose production in the liver and helping muscles and fat cells use insulin, and it decreases Hgb A1C by 1.5 to 2 percent. The most commonly seen adverse reaction with metformin is diarrhea (53.2 percent). Other common problems are nausea and vomiting (25.5 percent), flatulence (12.1 percent), indigestion (7.1 percent), and headache (5.7 percent).[15] A black box warning on metformin concerns lactic acidosis, a rare but serious metabolic complication that can occur because of metformin accumulation. Unfortunately, lactic acidosis is fatal in approximately 50 percent of cases. Lactic acidosis may also occur in association with a number of pathophysiologic conditions, including diabetes mellitus, and whenever there is significant lack of blood flow to an area or lack of oxygenation. Lactic acidosis is characterized by elevated blood lactate levels, which increase the body's acidity to dangerous levels.[16]

2. Cimetidine (Trade Name: Tagamet)

Cimetidine treats gastric ulcers, gastroesophageal reflux disease (GERD), and heartburn. The most common side effects are diarrhea, dizziness, drowsiness, and headache. Some patients can experience allergic reactions (causing anaphylaxis), fatigue, joint/muscle pain, or slow/fast heartbeat. This class of drugs, called H_2 antagonists, lowers acid amounts produced in the stomach. Another drug in this same class is the OTC famotidine (Pepcid).[17]

3. Alcohol (Ethyl Alcohol)

Alcohol is a recreational drink. Alcohol intoxication can result in abdominal pain, vomiting, blurred vision, and mental changes. When asked about their consumption of alcohol, the majority of people underestimate the amount actually consumed.[18] In the year 2004 61 percent of adults in the United States drank alcohol; 32 percent of those who drank reported drinking at least five drinks on at least one day over the year.[19]

LET'S RECAP

Patient: James, age 55
1. Metformin (Glucophage) for type 2 diabetes: 500 mg 2 times a day
2. Cimetidine (Tagamet) for heartburn: 200 mg
3. Alcohol (recreational): 1 whiskey sour and 1 beer 2 times a day

Lab-test results:
pH: 7.30 (normally 7.35–7.45)
Anion gap: 15 mM/L (normally 12 mM/L)
Bicarb: 18 mEq/L (normally 24–31 mEq/L)
SCr (serum creatinine): 1.6 mg/dL (normally 0.6–1.4 mg/dL)
Lactate: 6 mM/L (normally 0.5–1.0 mM/L)
X-ray findings: Not applicable

SUMMARY REPORT

An initial evaluation of the situation suggests that James's medical problems are not directly causing the symptoms and that the following information must be considered:

- Dr. Louie has just started James on metformin last week.

- Serum creatinine (SCr) is an indication of kidney function. James's SCr is a little high, which means his kidney function is lower than normal.

- The body's normal pH range is 7.35 to 7.45. James's pH is 7.35, which is on the low end of normal and means his body is in an acidic state.

- James's lactate level is high at 6 mM/L.

SOLVE THE MYSTERY

Hmmm, for a hint to solve the mystery, take another look at the lab-test results…the abnormal lab values for some tests are all related to a medication that was recently added.

The Culprit: Metformin-Induced Lactic Acidosis

The word *lactic* refers to lactate buildup, and the word *acidosis* refers to a pH lower than 7.35. Lactic acidosis is a rare but serious metabolic complication that can occur when metformin builds up in the blood during treatment. Lactic acidosis occurs because of the way metformin works. Metformin enhances anaerobic metabolism (metabolism without oxygen). A by-product of anaerobic metabolism is lactate; therefore, too much metformin could potentially cause too much lactate.

The onset of lactic acidosis is often subtle and accompanied only by nonspecific symptoms, such as fatigue, muscle pain, respiratory distress, increasing tiredness, and abdominal distress. Hypothermia, low blood pressure, and slowed heart rates may also be associated with this reaction. An easy way to think of the muscle pain is to remember a time when you may have worked too hard and a few hours later your muscles were very achy. When you work your muscles very hard, they don't get enough oxygen, and therefore not enough lactate is removed from the muscles. The pain and soreness is due to lactate buildup in your muscles. The same thing happens with lactic acidosis, except this condition affects your entire body.

Lactic acidosis is characterized by elevated blood lactate levels (5 mmol/L or more), decreased blood pH (<7.35), and increased anion gap (>12 mmol/L).[20]

The Accomplices: Alcohol, Cimetidine, COPD

It is important to evaluate the patient's concurrent medications, alcohol use, and diseases since all of these factors can increase the potential for an adverse drug reaction.

- Alcohol reduces the conversion of lactate to glucose. It also slows down the rate at which the liver can pull lactate out of the blood. Both actions can cause increased levels of lactate.

- Cimetidine slows down the removal of metformin from the body. When the two drugs are taken together, metformin's overall level can be increased up to 40 percent. And as stated previously, too much metformin could mean too much lactate.[21]

- Patients with COPD don't get oxygen to their organs and the rest of their body like a healthy patient would, so they are already predisposed to experiencing anaerobic metabolism (which produces lactate as a by-product).

THE SOLUTION

James got to the hospital just in time. Lactic acidosis is a serious condition that can be fatal in up to 50 percent of cases. After realizing that James had just started metformin a week earlier, Dr. Louie recognizes this could be the problem. He orders tests to check the lactate level, pH, and electrolytes in James's body to verify the diagnosis of lactic acidosis. After the lab results come back and confirm that diagnosis, Dr. Louie immediately tells James to stop taking his metformin and prescribes a different medication for his diabetes. James isn't too far gone, so after some supportive therapeutic measures and three days in the hospital, he is able to go home.[22]

WHAT ARE YOUR CHANCES?

The reported incidence of lactic acidosis in patients receiving metformin is very low (approximately 0.03 cases per 1,000 patient-years, with approximately 0.015 fatal cases per 1,000 patient-years).[23] More than twenty thousand patient-years of exposure to metformin have been documented in clinical trials, and lactic acidosis was not observed. The FDA estimates that 5 out of 100,000 people will acquire lactic acidosis at any time during their treatment on metformin.[24]

The patients who are at the highest risk of lactic acidosis have other physical problems. The most common risk factor is kidney failure, because if the kidneys aren't working right, metformin doesn't leave the body as it should. Other problems are congestive heart failure, because the heart can't pump enough blood (and therefore oxygen), and any other disease that compromises the lungs (such as COPD, emphysema, lung cancer, or pneumonia). (36,786,000 Rxs/12 Rxs per patient-year = 3,065,500 patient-years × 0.03 per 1,000 patient-years = 92 cases/year.) In 2007 105 cases of metformin-induced lactic acidosis were reported to the FDA's MedWatch database.[25] This is quite a large number of reported cases to the FDA. Metformin-induced lactic acidosis is a real risk for patients, and it is important to remember that if you have a disease that increases your risk for lactic acidosis, you should be leery of starting treatment with metformin.

This reaction is an extremely rare reaction to metformin therapy. The reaction almost exclusively occurs in patients with decreased kidney function. Your physician should have your blood frequently tested to evaluate your kidney function to decrease the risk of this reaction occurring. However, with only ninety-two estimated cases out of more than three million patients, patients who follow their schedules for lab tests should not have to worry about this complication.[26] James did not follow Rule #6, which could have prevented a hospitalization. Also, Rule #10 could have alerted him to the importance of not consuming alcohol with metformin. Alcohol increases the risk for lactic acidosis and should not be consumed while on metformin.

Overall, metformin is pretty safe, especially in the case of lactic acidosis; it doesn't occur that often. However, it is important not to drink alcoholic beverages while you are taking metformin. If you do drink alcohol, limit yourself to one or two beverages a week. More than that causes concerns about the liver's ability to adequately clear enough lactate from your body to keep you safe.

Also, it is important to remember that metformin is contraindicated in kidney failure. That means it absolutely should never be used if your kidneys are not working, because the lactate could build up and cause toxicities. Kidney function is usually measured by a parameter called SCr (serum creatinine), and normally this number is around 1 mg/dL. Do not use metforin if your SCr levels are in the ranges shown below:

Populations for Which Metformin Is Contraindicated

- men with a SCr level > 1.5 mg/dL
- women with a SCr level > 1.4 mg/dL

If doctors ever talk to you about kidney failure, make sure they know you're on metformin and you may need to be taken off this drug, depending on your SCr level.

You should not be on metformin if you have significant hepatic (liver-related) disease, alcoholism, and any disease that may increase hypoxia (low oxygen levels), such as COPD. Many situations can predispose you to lactic acidosis. If you become dehydrated, do not take your next dose of metformin, because dehydration increases your chances of lactic acidosis. Elderly patients need to have their kidney function checked on schedule. Just being older can increase the risks of lactic acidosis. Do not take metformin forty-eight hours before a medical procedure. You can begin taking it again once you are eating and drinking normally. Doses above 1.7 g/day, especially if you are elderly or have mild renal (kidney) dysfunction, can greatly increase your risk of lactic acidosis.[27]

 ### VIOLATION OF RULE #6: Know Your Lab-Test Schedule

Before you start taking metformin, you should have your kidneys checked to make sure they are functioning properly. Have your serum creatinine (SCr) levels checked and then rechecked every three months to make sure your body can remove the lactate that is produced. At home, if you notice any signs of unusual muscle pain, labored breathing, abnormally slow heart rate, or progressive fatigue, contact your doctor immediately. Time is very important when treating lactic acidosis. Reports state that up to 50 percent of patients with lactic acidosis die. That is a big number! Don't miss appointments to have your kidney lab values checked

 ### VIOLATION OF RULE #10: Understand That Over-the-Counter Medicines, Herbals, and Alcohol Are All Drugs

If James had read the patient information regarding metformin, he would have noticed that he should limit his alcohol intake. Alcohol is a drug, and if you're not careful, alcohol can have serious effects while you're on metformin. Had James limited his intake of alcohol, along with more closely watching his kidney function, he may have been able to prevent this reaction.

Medication-Induced Hypoglycemia (Low Blood Sugar)

The following case shows us that some medications can cause hypoglycemia, a condition that indicates low blood glucose.

THE PATIENT

Ed, or "Mr. Ed," as the young kids on the block call him, is a forty-eight-year-old widower who lives alone but down the block from his daughter and son-in-law. He is overweight (230 lb.), has high blood pressure, and is an insulin-dependent type 2 diabetic. Ed is embarrassed about his diabetes and injects his insulin before his daughter comes over. Ed is a "supernice guy," but lately his daughter has been noticing some weird mood changes in Ed, and she's afraid he's actually losing his mind.

THE SYMPTOMS

Ed's daughter comes over for lunch about three times a week to make sure he's eating healthy food and has something good to eat for dinner. For about the last month, though, right before lunch, Ed always seems to be really confused. He has called her by the wrong name and tries to watch TV shows that are only on at night. He once even tries to walk the dog, but the dog passed away eight years ago. She has also noticed that he's not walking very well; he has been holding on to walls, and she catches him once when he almost falls. He's also consistently sweaty, shaky, and really kind of crabby before lunch. He's only forty-eight years old, though, and she can't imagine what is wrong with him.

THE SUSPECTS

The likely suspects are the following drugs.

1. Aspirin (Trade Names: Bayer, Ecotrin, Ascriptin, Bufferin, Easprin, St. Joseph Adult Aspirin)

Aspirin treats pain and fever and reduces the risk of death in heart attack and strokes by decreasing platelet clotting. It can cause nausea, vomiting, and dizziness.[28]

The chemical structure name is acetylsalicylic acid (ASA), and this drug is in the subclass of salicylates that can cause Reye's syndrome in children (see http://www.healthline.com/adamcontent /reye-syndrome for more information). Aspirin is a nonsteroidal anti inflammatory drug (NSAID), and taking it with other NSAIDs may decrease platelet effect, which means doing so can lead to less blood clotting and a higher risk of bleeding. Ed is taking it because he has two cardiovascular risk factors: high blood pressure and obesity. Because age is also a risk factor, taking an aspirin is recommended for men who are at least fifty years of age or older.[29]

2. Insulin Regular (Trade Name: Humulin R)

Humulin R is used for the treatment of type 1 and type 2 diabetes mellitus that is unresponsive to treatment with diet and/or oral hypoglycemics (which decrease blood sugars) to control hyperglycemia (high blood sugars). It replaces the insulin that the body should be making in response to meals. Side effects of this medication include hypoglycemia (low blood sugar); mental confusion; rapid heartbeat; paleness; fatigue; headache; itching, redness, pain, or warmth at the injection site; hunger; nausea; and hypokalemia (low potassium).

It is a short-acting insulin that is usually taken before meals and as needed for high blood sugar. Typically, it lasts between six and eight hours, and the time to onset (that is, the amount of time that elapses before it starts to lower blood sugar) is approximately thirty minutes. Injection is usually made into the abdomen, thighs, arms, or buttocks, and it is important to rotate among these sites. Cold injections of insulin should be avoided, because they are more likely to sting or to be painful.[30]

3. Insulin Glargine (Trade Name: Lantus)

Lantus is used for the treatment of type 1 and type 2 diabetes mellitus that is unresponsive to treatment with diet and/or oral hypoglycemics (which decrease blood sugars) to control hyperglycemia (high blood sugars). It replaces the baseline amount of insulin the body needs to survive. Side effects include hypoglycemia (low blood sugar); mental confusion; rapid heartbeat; paleness; fatigue; headache; itching, redness, pain, or warmth at the injection site; hunger; nausea; and hypokalemia (low potassium). Lantus is a long-acting insulin that provides twenty-four-hour coverage. This medication is injected once daily into the abdomen, usually at bedtime.[31]

LET'S RECAP

Patient: Ed, age 48

1. Aspirin to reduce risk of death by heart attack: 81 mg daily
2. Humulin R (insulin regular) for diabetes: 70 units before each meal daily
3. Lantus (insulin glargine) for diabetes (baseline insulin requirements): 30 units subcutaneously every night at bedtime

Lab-test results:

    Fasting blood sugar (FBS): 77 mg/dL (normally <100 mg/dL)

    Glucometer readings: 64, 75, 53, 46 mg/dL (before meals normally 90–130 mg/dL; 1–2 hours after the start of a meal normally less than 180 mg/dL; hypoglycemia if less than 70 mg/dL)

X-ray findings: Not applicable

SUMMARY REPORT

An initial evaluation of the situation suggests that Ed's health conditions are not directly causing the symptoms and that the following information must be considered:

- Ed has always been embarrassed about needing insulin and usually gives himself his shot before his daughter gets to his house.
- A normal fasting blood sugar (FBS) is less than 100 mg/dL.
- A goal FBS for diabetics is less than 126 mg/dL.

- Normal glucose levels in diabetics should be:
  - before meals = 90 to 130 mg/dL
  - 1–2 hours after start of meal = less than 180 mg/dL
  - hypoglycemia = 70 mg/dL or below
- A normal dose of insulin is 0.5 to 1 unit/kg/day. This is only a guideline and certainly can be increased in patients who are insulin-resistant.

SOLVE THE MYSTERY

Take a closer look at Ed's lab-test results after you read the clues. His blood sugar is extremely low. What medication is causing the low blood sugar? The aspirin wouldn't affect blood sugar; it is an anti-inflammatory, antiplatelet medication. But wow, look at that dose of Humulin R (insulin regular).

The Culprit: Insulin-Induced Hypoglycemia

As stated in the clues, the normal dose of insulin is 0.5 to 1 unit/kg/day. Ed is taking 70 units before each meal, so that's 210 units per day. Now he weighs 230 lbs., and that's 105 kg. Doing the math:

210 units / 105 kg = 2 units/kg/day

Some people may have to go up as high as 2 units/kg/day, but not Ed. His blood sugar is certainly too low; in fact, all his readings are in the hypoglycemic range. Hypoglycemia causes hunger, nervousness, shakiness, perspiration, dizziness, sleepiness, confusion, difficulty speaking, and an anxious or weak feeling,[32] so no wonder he is feeling so poorly.

The Accomplice: Time

Because Ed is embarrassed to give himself the shots, he always injects his insulin before his daughter arrives at his house. Consequently, he is letting too much time go by between taking the insulin shot and eating. Regular insulin works within fifteen to thirty minutes. That means the body is expecting some sugar (food) to deal with in the next half hour. If a person takes insulin but then doesn't eat within a half hour, they will almost always become hypoglycemic.[33]

THE SOLUTION

Ed's daughter makes an appointment for him to see the doctor in the following week. The doctor takes one look at Ed's glucose-meter readings and says, "Wow, Ed, I don't know how you've been getting around at all. We need to take your insulin way down." The doctor tells Ed to decrease his insulin (Humulin R) to 40 units before meals (1.2 units/kg/day) and to decrease his nighttime insulin (Lantus) to 25 units. He also tells Ed about the importance of eating within thirty minutes of taking his insulin. Lastly, Ed still has to test his sugar at least three times daily, before meals and then again once at bedtime.

Ed's doctor also makes him aware of the signs of hypoglycemia and how to react to the readings on his blood-glucose meter. If he has a reading below 70 mg/dL, he now knows to eat a "quick-fix" food.[34]

HELPFUL ADVICE

Hypoglycemia is exceedingly common in diabetics who are on insulin therapy. Every patient starting on insulin or any drug that may induce hypoglycemia should be educated about the signs and symptoms of hypoglycemia and how to successfully treat an episode. Increased risk of hypoglycemia can be due to several risk factors, such as advanced age, renal or hepatic dysfunction, a high dose of a drug that may cause hypoglycemia, decreased carbohydrate intake, drug interactions, hospitalization within the past thirty days, and recent alcohol use.[35] Strive to be aware of your risks and ways to avoid an adverse reaction when taking any medication. Ed has violated Rules #1 and #7. Always recognize insulin as a potentially dangerous drug if not taken properly and know your monitoring parameters (the measurement of the effectiveness of the medication).

Signs and symptoms of hypoglycemia can vary from person to person. Some symptoms that may warn you that your sugar is getting too low include nausea, weakness/fatigue, confusion, blurred vision, irritability, feeling cold or clammy, nervousness, and a rapid heartbeat. Get to know your own signs, and describe them to your friends and family so they will be able to help you. If you take insulin or a diabetes medication that can cause hypoglycemia, always carry one of the quick-fix foods with you. Wearing a medical identification bracelet or necklace is also a good idea.[36]

Exercise can also cause hypoglycemia. Check your blood glucose before you exercise. Also, eating a pre-exercise snack can help prevent low blood sugar readings. Severe hypoglycemia can cause you to lose consciousness. In these extreme cases when you lose consciousness and cannot eat a snack to bring your blood sugar back up, glucagon can be injected to quickly raise your blood glucose level. Make sure your doctor provides you with one of these kits.

Also of note is the newer concept of taking diabetes-education classes. Certified diabetes educators are nurses and pharmacists specifically trained to educate diabetic patients on managing their diabetes on their own. They are able to provide many specific details regarding how diabetes affects your body, signs and symptoms to recognize whether you have high or low blood sugar, glucose meter instruction, insulin injection instruction, and a multitude of other educational information. They also tend to offer diet counseling sessions to help you eat a balanced diet that reduces your blood sugar but keeps it level. Dieticians are a valuable resource for any diabetic patient. You may also want to take a family member with you to help them realize the problems you may face with your diabetes. If you are worried about the costs associated with diabetes-education classes, many insurance plans, including Medicare, pay for some or all of the associated costs. Take advantage of this opportunity.

VIOLATION OF RULE #1: Learn from Others—What Is Happening in the ER?

The use and misuse of insulin is one of the most common reasons patients show up at the emergency room. Had Ed realized this problem, he may have been more cautious with his insulin injections. Also, simple use of a glucose meter would have alerted Ed and his physician earlier that he was having problems with his glucose control. Ed did not know what the numbers meant and was concerned about the stigma of insulin injections. This embarrassment cost Ed a trip to the emergency room. Proper teaching about how to use insulin and a glucose meter is vital. Many patients go too low on their insulin injections and manage their diabetes poorly, causing them to fall, have racing heartbeats, or experience increased sweating, fatigue, and loss of consciousness. However, insulin is a necessary medication for many diabetics; therefore, it is vital to use this medication correctly.

VIOLATION OF RULE #7: Know Your Medication's Monitoring Parameters

Patients need to be aware of proper monitoring techniques for blood sugar and what to do about them when readings are outside the recommended range. Your blood sugar should be tested at least three times a day, especially when you feel the symptoms of hypoglycemia. This helps you adequately correct your low blood sugar in time and ensures that you maintain your optimal diabetic sugar levels. The best option for a diabetic patient, whether newly diagnosed or a diabetic for twenty-plus years, is to sign up with a certified diabetes educator for classes on diabetes management.

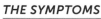

CONDITION

Medication-Induced Stevens-Johnson Syndrome (a Painful Rash That Spreads and Blisters Like a Burn)

The following case shows us that some medications can cause Stevens-Johnson Syndrome, also known as erythema multiforme major, a condition in which the skin and mucous membranes react severely to a medication or infection, resulting in a painful red or purplish rash that spreads and blisters like a burn.

THE PATIENT

Luke has just gotten back from a fourteen-day medical mission trip to Colombia. He is a twenty-three-year-old medical student who is out to save the world. He's very healthy, eats well, exercises, and has no health problems to speak of. He does drink about a gallon of coffee every day and takes ginseng daily, too. However, the day after he returns to the United States, he starts having five to six loose, watery stools a day. He also has nausea, vomiting, abdominal cramping, and a fever. He goes to the doctor, and she confirms what he suspects: Luke has traveler's diarrhea. The doctor starts him on Bactrim (sulfamethoxazole/trimethoprim) 160/800 mg twice a day for the next five days.[37]

THE SYMPTOMS

The next day, Luke starts to feel really bad. He is worried he may have caught the flu along with the traveler's diarrhea. He still has a fever, but now he has a bad headache and chills, and he is coughing up some pretty gross stuff. The day after that, he notices a strange rash on his stomach and the palms of his hands. It looks like a bunch of little circles on his belly, with dark spots on the insides. They almost resemble little targets. He thinks this is pretty strange, especially because it appears on his palms. He goes back to the doctor, and she tells him he is lucky he came in so soon. She calls an ambulance and gets Luke hospitalized immediately.[38]

THE SUSPECTS

The likely suspects are the following drugs.

1. Caffeine

Caffeine is a central nervous system (CNS) stimulant that wakes up the brain. It can cause increased heart rate, cardiac arrhythmia, insomnia, nervousness, muscular tremor, headache, nausea, vomiting, and stomach pain. It is possible to overdose on caffeine, which would cause cardiac arrhythmia or seizure. Most people experience withdrawal symptoms if their bodies become used to a certain amount of caffeine per day and this amount is suddenly decreased. Even though a doctor's prescription isn't required to obtain it, caffeine is still a drug.[39]

2. Ginseng

Although it has no FDA indication for treatment of disease, ginseng has been used for multiple reasons, including but not limited to increasing the mental and physical capacity for work and protecting against diabetes. The most common side effects are nervousness and excitation. It has been shown to interact with furosemide, nifedipine, and warfarin. As with caffeine, even though a prescription isn't needed to obtain it, ginseng is still a drug.[40]

3. Sulfamethoxazole/Trimethoprim (Trade Name: Bactrim)

Sulfamethoxazole/trimethoprim treats bacterial infections due to *E. coli, Klebsiella, Enterobacter, M. morganii, P. mirabilis, P. vulgaris, Shigella enteritis, Pneumocystis carinii pneumonia, H. influenzae,* and *S. pneumoniae.* Side effects include allergic reactions, hypersensitivity of the respiratory tract, Stevens-Johnson Syndrome (SJS), toxic epidermal necrolysis, megaloblastic anemia due to folate deficiency, and increased amount of adverse reactions in elderly patients. It is a sulfa-based antibiotic, so patients with a known sulfa allergy should avoid taking it.[41]

LET'S RECAP

Patient: Luke, age 23

1. Sulfamethoxazole/trimethoprim (Bactrim) 160/800 mg for traveler's diarrhea: 1 tablet 2 times daily for 5 days
2. Caffeine as a CNS stimulant: 100 mg 3 times daily
3. Ginseng extract as a physical and mental stimulation: 300 mg daily

Lab-test results:

SCr (serum creatinine): 1.2 mg/L (normally 0.6–1.4 mg/L)

WBC (white blood count): 12,000 cells/mL (normally 4,500–10,000 cells/mL)

Temp: 101°F (normally 98.6°F)

Blood pressure: 96/61 mmHg (normally 120/80 mmHg)

HR: 115 bpm (normally 60–100 bpm)

Other tests:

Skin biopsy: Epidermal cell necrosis with lymphocytes present

SUMMARY REPORT

An initial evaluation of the situation suggests that no particular disease is causing the symptoms and that the following information must be considered:

- Luke's hand has circular lesions with a target-like appearance. The "targets" have dark centers, or bull's-eyes, of dead tissue. Targetlike lesions cover both his hands and his abdomen, too. This rash is indicative of SJS.

- Luke also has a slight fever and an elevated white blood cell count, which are signs of infection.

- His blood pressure is a little low, and his heart rate is a little high. These are signs that his vital signs (blood pressure, heart rate) are unstable, which means he is in danger of having negative outcomes, such as sepsis (infection in the blood).

- Lastly, the results of his skin biopsy confirm SJS.[42]

SOLVE THE MYSTERY

Luke, unfortunately, has been diagnosed with SJS. This particular kind of rash has one of four causes: infection, drugs, cancer, or idiopathy (meaning the cause is unknown). We know he's recently been out of the country, which means we have to be on the lookout for uncommon bacteria and viruses, but first let's check out his medications.[43]

The Culprit: Bactrim-Induced Stevens-Johnson Syndrome

As stated, Bactrim has a number of side effects, and one of the most serious is SJS. SJS is an immune hypersensitivity reaction, meaning that the patient's immune system overacts and attacks the body. SJS typically involves the skin and the mucous membranes. Mucosa is the tissue that lines body passages for communication, either directly or indirectly with the exterior. It functions to protect, to support, and to absorb nutrients, along with secreting mucus, enzymes, and electrolytes.

Examples of affected areas are the inside of the mouth, inside of the nose, lining of the eyes, genital mucosa, GI tract, or lower respiratory mucosa.

TYPICAL PROGRESSION OF STEVENS-JOHNSON SYNDROME

1. SJS starts with purulent cough (one containing pus), headache, fatigue, and joint pain that lasts one to fourteen days.
2. An abrupt outbreak of skin lesions occurs.
   a. Lesions typically look like targets, with the centermost dark spot being dead skin.
   b. The dead skin sloughs off, leaving parts of the body unprotected.
   c. Lesions can occur anywhere but are common on the palms and soles of the hands, the abdomen, and the mucosa.
3. Patients must be hospitalized until the outbreak of lesions stops. They are typically treated as burn victims, because the sloughed-off skin leaves their bodies unprotected.
4. Infection is a common problem because of the areas of the body unprotected by skin.

The term *SJS* is sometimes confused with the term *toxic epidermal necrolysis (TEN)*. The only difference between the terms is the percentage of the body affected.

- SJS affects less than 10 percent of body surface area (BSA).
- SJS/TEN affects 10 to 30 percent of BSA.
- TEN affects greater than 30 percent of BSA.

Morbidity (Complications)

- Lesions may continue to erupt for two to three weeks.
- Complications of lesions may include:
  - infection
  - scarring
  - narrowing of the esophagus
  - respiratory failure (mucus shedding in the respiratory tract)
  - blindness in 3 to 10 percent of patients because of eye mucosa damage
  - vaginal narrowing and penile scarring

Mortality

- determined by extent of skin sloughing
- affected BSA < 10 percent = mortality rate of 1 to 5 percent
- affected BSA ≥ 30 percent = mortality rate of 25 to 35 percent[11]

THE SOLUTION

Luke is very lucky, because he and his doctor catch the problem early and he stops taking the sulfamethoxazole/trimethoprim (Bactrim). Better outcomes have been linked to early diagnosis. He is immediately sent to the hospital, where medical staff watch and wait to see how his disease progresses. In his case, the lesions on his abdomen erupt for about two weeks, but he never has skin sloughing in more than 10 percent of his BSA. He does suffer from lesions and cell sloughing in his mouth, which makes eating very painful.

He is treated with intravenous fluids to counteract dehydration, good wound care to stop infection, numbing mouthwashes and topical agents, and pain control. He stays in the hospital for nineteen days.

Luke is also incredibly lucky that his wounds never become infected. That is partially due to good hospital care: constant hand washing, vigilant staff, and expert wound care. It is also due to his being young and otherwise healthy.[45]

WHAT ARE YOUR CHANCES?

Based on 2006 data presented in the *Journal of American Medicine,* sulfonamide-containing antibiotics accounted for 2.2 percent of all visits to the emergency room because of adverse drug reactions. This translates into 15,593 emergency-room visits due to reactions to sulfa antibiotics.

However, this does not mean that 15,593 people had SJS. The majority of the emergency-room visits were due to high-risk patients—that is, elderly patients with liver or kidney disease, or patients with HIV.

In fact, an estimated 1 to 3 in 100,000 users of sulfamethoxazole/trimethoprim (Bactrim) will get SJS. That is a relatively low estimate, especially in comparison to some other drugs. For example, carbamazepine (trade name Tegretol) is an anticonvulsant with a chance of SJS that is 14 in 100,000 users. Nevertheless, if you are taking sulfamethoxazole/trimethoprim, be aware that SJS is a potentially lethal side effect, and be on the lookout for the characteristic rash. (8,335,000 Rxs × 1–3 percent incidence = 83,350–250,050 cases/year.) Eleven cases of SJS were reported to the FDA's Med-Watch system in 2007.[46] The low incidence of reported cases does not mean that the risk for SJS isn't present.[47]

HELPFUL ADVICE

SJS is another rare reaction for the typical patient. However, any rash as a result of drug therapy should be immediately investigated. Many drugs have been associated with SJS, and this condition should not be ignored if a problem arises. The most common drugs for SJS are antibiotics (sulfa, such as sulfamethoxazole/trimethoprim, penicillins, and cephalosporins), antiepileptics (carbemazepine, phenytoin, lamotrigine, and phenobarbital), antigout medications (allopurinol), and NSAIDs (piroxicam).[48] (For a full list of the medication classes that can cause SJS see the table below.)

Medication or Medication Class Associated with SJS[49]*

Medication Class	Examples
Allopurinol	Zyloprim (antigout)
Aminopenicillins	Amoxicillin, Amoxil, Augmentin (antibiotics)
Carbamazepine	Tegretol, (antiepileptic)
Cephalosporins	Keflex, Ceftin (antibiotics)
Corticosteroids	Prednisone, prednisolone
Oxicam NSAIDs	Feldene, Piroxicam
Phenobarbital	(antiepileptic)
Phenytoin	Dilantin (antiepileptic)
Quinolones	Levaquin, Avelox, Cipro (antibiotics)
Sulfa drugs	Sulfamethoxazole/trimethoprim
Valproic acid	Depakote (antiepileptic)

* Adapted from J. C. Roujeau et al, "Medication Use and the Risk of Stevens-Johnson Syndrome or Toxic Epidermal Necrolysis," in *New England Journal of Medicine* 333, no. 24 (1995): 1600–1607. http://www.nejm.org/doi/full/10.1056 /NEJM199512143332404.

Tips for Recognizing Drug-Induced Rashes

Rashes are tricky. Nine times out of ten, you think you have something serious, and it just turns out to be irritation from a new lotion or something equally harmless. However, that one exception could be something serious, so it is always important to keep track of your rash. To help you out, here are some generalized rules.[50]

1. If the Rash Is Troubling You, Go See Your Doctor.

At the end of the day, it is your body and your skin, and if you are worried about a rash, have it checked out. It may be treatable with an over-the-counter product, but if you don't know what it is, you can't treat it.

2. The Longer You've Had a Rash, the More Likely It Is You Should Have a Doctor Check It Out.

Most of the time, a rash that has been present for a couple of days will go away on its own. However, some warning signs, such as pain, rapid swelling causing shortness of breath, bleeding blisters in the mouth or eyes, skin that is rapidly turning dusky or black, and large amounts of skin peeling in sheets, indicate that you should see the doctor sooner rather than later.

3. If You've Had the Same Rash Before, the Diagnosis Is Probably the Same.

This may sound oversimplified, but many people think that because a rash comes back, it wasn't diagnosed correctly. Actually, many rashes aren't necessarily cured but controlled. Some rashes, such as eczema, atopic dermatitis, seborrheic dermatitis, psoriasis, hives, and rosacea, can come and go depending on many factors. The best idea is to educate yourself about a rash you've been diagnosed with so you know what to expect in the future. You may be surprised to find out you need to continue some type of treatment to keep it under control.

 VIOLATION OF RULE #11: If Your Health Changes after You Add a New Drug, Think Drug-Induced Disease

Luke initially thought his symptoms meant he had the flu, so he did not consider the possibility that the new prescription for Bactrim could be the culprit. In addition, SJS is an example of a life-threatening adverse drug reaction that just happens. Certain medications are more likely to cause such a rash; however, no one can predict which patients will develop the rash. No rhyme or reason predisposes patients to the severe rash presented with SJS. As a patient, your best option is to recognize a rash and immediately contact your physician or pharmacist. If you have reason to believe that a rash is due to a drug, stop taking that medication and contact your doctor immediately. Time is very important in treating SJS: The earlier you recognize the infamous target patterns typical of this type of rash, the better your chances of survival. Know what to look for, and know the common offenders. This problem will likely never affect you or anyone you know, but it could, so it is important to recognize the signs and symptoms to be prepared should the need arise.

▆▆▆▆▆ CONDITION ▆▆▆▆▆

Medication-Induced Rhabdomyolysis (Muscle Pain)

The following case shows us that some medications can cause rhabdomyolysis. Rhabdomyolysis is the breakdown of skeletal muscle.

THE PATIENT

Kyle is a thirty-nine-year-old accountant who decides this year that his New Year's resolution is to get into shape and to be healthy. He starts an exercise program, adds fruits and vegetables to his diet, and visits his doctor for a routine physical. Kyle is already taking medication for high cholesterol and depression/anxiety. His doctor decides his cholesterol level isn't as good as it could be and adds a medication called gemfibrozil to help lower his triglycerides.

THE SYMPTOMS

About a month into the New Year's resolution plans, Kyle starts to notice that his back and legs are just really achy, almost like he has just run a marathon. He initially thinks the pain results from the exercise program he has started, but then he realizes he hasn't actually been to the gym in two weeks because he has been so tired lately. He spends about another week just thinking he has the flu, but he isn't coughing, and he doesn't have any fevers or chills. He tells his pharmacist about his troubles when he goes to refill his medications, and his pharmacist tells him to make an appointment with his doctor to talk about the possibility that his medications are making him sick. The next day, he attends his appointment with his physician. The doctor cannot figure out why Kyle's legs are so weak, so he decides to admit Kyle to the hospital to run some tests.

THE SUSPECTS

The likely suspects are the following drugs.

1. Simvastatin (Trade Name: Zocor)

Simvastatin lowers LDL ("bad") cholesterol and triglyceride levels and raises HDL ("good") cholesterol. It can also cause muscle pain (<1 percent), rhabdomyolysis with acute renal failure secondary to myoglobinuria (<1 percent), raised liver enzyme levels (AST [aspartate aminotransferase], ALT [alanine transaminase], LDH [lactate dehydrogenase], bilirubin, and Alk Phos [alkaline phosphatase] in 1 percent), abdominal pain (1–3 percent), and nausea (1 percent). This medication is a statin like Lipitor (atorvastatin).[51]

2. Gemfibrozil (Trade Name: Lopid)

Gemfibrozil lowers serum triglyceride levels and increases HDLs and is usually used in patients whose triglycerides are very high. Side effects include gallstones (7.5 percent vs. 4.9 percent for the placebo group, a 55 percent excess for the gemfibrozil group), muscle pain, raised liver enzymes (AST, ALT, LDH, bilirubin, and Alk Phos), and GI reactions (34.2 percent vs. 23.8 percent on placebo). This medication is a fibrate, meaning it works by limiting the breakdown of fat stores and decreasing the amounts of fatty acids the liver takes from food. Both of these actions work to decrease triglycerides.[52]

3. Citalopram (Trade Name: Celexa)

Citalopram is most commonly used to treat depression, but it can also be used for obsessive-compulsive disorder (OCD), panic disorder, generalized anxiety, and posttraumatic stress. It is a selective serotonin reuptake inhibitor (SSRI). The most common side effects of this medication are nausea (7 percent), somnolence (8 percent), and sexual dysfunction (3–5 percent). Irritability, insomnia, and headache are possible if treatment is abruptly discontinued. Citalopram carries a black box warning stating that the risk of suicide increases in children and adolescents. It should not be used with monoamine oxidase inhibitors (MAOIs) because of the potential for serotonin syndrome. (MAOIs, such as Marplan, Nardil, Parnate, Emsam, or Azilect, are monoamine oxidase inhibitors, a strong class of medications used for treating depression.)[53]

LET'S RECAP

Patient: Kyle, age 39
1. Simvastatin (Zocor) for high cholesterol: 40 mg daily
2. Gemfibrozil (Lopid) for high triglycerides: 600 mg 2 times daily
3. Citalopram (Celexa) for depression/anxiety: 20 mg daily
Lab-test results:
    LDL: 137 mg/dL (normally <100 mg/dL)
    HDL: 46 mg/dL (normally >40 mg/dL)
    TG (triglycerides): 543 mg/dL (normally <150 mg/dL)
    CK (creatinine kinase): 1,700 IU/L (normally 72–198 IU/L)
    SCr (serum creatinine): 2.6 mg/dL (normally 0.6–1.4 mg/dL)
    Urine myoglobin: Positive
X-ray findings: Not applicable

SUMMARY REPORT

An initial evaluation of the situation suggests that Kyle's health conditions are not directly causing the symptoms he is experiencing and that the following information must be considered:

- Signs of myopathy and rhabdomyolysis:

  1. creatinine kinase (CK) >170 IU/L

  2. urine positive for myoglobin

  3. SCr >1 mg/dL

  4. positive muscle symptoms (weakness and pain)

- Co-administration of gemfibrozil and simvastatin resulted in an increase in the amount of simvastatin in the body by 185 percent.

- When given together, the dose of simvastatin should not exceed 10 mg/day.[54]

SOLVE THE MYSTERY

Muscle pain and an elevated CK (creatinine kinase) are the classic signs of statin-induced myopathy. The muscle pain is usually felt all over, but especially in the lower back and legs. Because Kyle hasn't worked out in a while, and we know that taking simvastatin and gemfibrozil together can cause myopathy and rhabdomyolysis, the culprit obviously is…[55]

The Culprits: Simvastatin- and Gemfibrozil-Induced Rhabdomyolysis

Kyle has been taking simvastatin for a while before his doctor adds gemfibrozil. Even if the gemfibrozil had not been added, Kyle still could have gotten rhabdomyolysis—it is just not as likely.

Fact: The average length of time a patient is on a statin before rhabdomyolysis occurs is about one year.

Fact: After adding a fibrate to a statin, the average time before rhabdomyolysis occurs is thirty-two days.

Drivers take considerable caution when approaching dangerous intersections that are known to be the common site of accidents. This same idea applies to medications. Taking statins and fibrates together increases the risk of rhabdomyolysis more than taking either medication alone. A "caution sign" should pop into the head of anyone approaching this dangerous intersection of medications.

The exact method by which statins and fibrates cause rhabdomyolysis is unclear. We know that statins work by decreasing the amount of cholesterol the liver makes. We think that reducing the amount of cholesterol in the body hurts the muscles in one of the following three ways:

1. It causes dysfunction in cell membranes.

2. It negatively affects the way cells obtain oxygen.

3. It disrupts the way a cell functions by interfering with protein messaging.

The end result of rhabdomyolysis is muscle breakdown. Parts of the muscle (myoglobin) are then excreted in the kidneys, which can cause serious kidney damage. The muscle symptoms will disappear and other lab readings will return to normal after the medication is stopped, but the kidney damage could cause long-term problems if not treated promptly.[56]

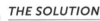 *The Accomplice: Gemfibrozil*

As stated earlier, taking gemfibrozil and simvastatin together increases the total amount of simvastatin by approximately 185 percent. Also, when a person is on both medications, the simvastatin dose should not be greater than 10 mg per day, and Kyle is on 40 mg.[57]

THE SOLUTION

Kyle stops taking the simvastatin and the gemfibrozil. Kyle also needs to get intravenous fluids in the hospital to help his kidneys flush out all the myoglobin in his blood. He stays in the hospital and receives supportive care until his kidney function returns to normal (as indicated by a SCr level of approximately 1 mg/dL.)

Once patients have myopathy or rhabdomyolysis, they are more likely to get it again if they ever go back on a statin. But Kyle's cholesterol numbers aren't very good, and that puts him at risk for a heart attack, among other things. So he's really going to have to focus on diet and exercise to help get his cholesterol level down. Maybe after some time has passed his doctor might try a low dose of a statin again, with extremely close monitoring, but that is only if the doctor thinks the benefits of low cholesterol outweigh the risk of myopathy and rhabdomyolysis.[58]

WHAT ARE YOUR CHANCES?

Muscle pain and weakness (myopathy) are more common than rhabdomyolysis. Depending on which statin you take, myopathies occur in 0.5 to 3 percent of all patients. Statins are associated with 0.1 to 7 percent in patients on a single drug and an incidence of 0.5 to 2.5 percent in patients using combination therapy. Studies have shown that lovastatin and simvastatin are associated with more myopathies than any other statin.[59] Many incidences of myopathies in statins are unknown; however, a few are known, including atorvastatin (3 percent), lovastatin (0.1–0.2 percent), pravastatin (0.1–0.2 percent), and simvastatin (2–7 percent).[60] Rhabdomyolysis is much less common, but your chances increase about tenfold if you're also on a fibrate. (47,174,000 Rxs for both simvastatin and gemfibrozil/ 12 Rxs per patient-year = 3,931,167 patient-years × 0.2062 percent = 8,106 cases of rhabdomyolysis/year, assuming everyone is on combination therapy.) (See the table below for information on how often rhabdomyolysis occurs with different medications.)

Incidence Rates of Rhabdomyolysis[61]

Medications that can cause rhabdomyolysis	Incidence rate per 1 year of therapy
Statins alone	0.0042 percent
Fibrates alone	0.0282 percent
Statin + fibrate	0.2062 percent

According to the FDA MedWatch reporting system for 2007, ninety-three cases of rhabdomyolysis were reported with simvastatin.[62] That is a large number of patients. Unfortunately, the FDA's system does not allow users to cross-reference those patients to identify who is on simvastatin *and* a fibrate, such as gemfibrozil.

HELPFUL ADVICE

Muscle aches and pain are commonly associated with statin therapy, but you need to be aware of the risks of rhabdomyolysis and alert your doctor to any symptoms that may indicate this complication. This is a major problem being seen in hospitals and can lead to serious complications if not discovered early. I've seen two cases of rhabdomyolysis in the same day, both due to the patients' being on a statin combined with gemfibrozil (Lopid) or Tricor. If you are on these medications and are feeling any aches and pains, see your doctor to have your CK levels evaluated. Rhabdomyolysis is rare, but people at risk should take it seriously. The drug manufacturers offer no information regarding the incidence of these occurrences, so it is important for you to know that these events are occurring in hospitals, and the possibility of it happening to you should be closely monitored.[63]

You should always do a number of things when you're taking a statin:

1. Be aware that if you experience muscle pain or weakness that you can't attribute to exercise or illness, your statin might be causing it.

2. Have your liver enzymes tested. Abnormal liver enzymes don't correlate to myopathy or rhabdomyolysis, but statins have the potential to raise liver enzyme levels, which is an indication of liver damage.

3. Know your lab values and track them over time. An increase in creatinine kinase (CK) in addition to symptoms of muscle weakness will alert the doctor to stop the medication. The creatinine kinase will then be retested, and the patient should be asked if the muscle weakness has improved.

4. Remind your doctor to get your lipid panel and your liver enzyme tests at least every six months when you're on statin meds, and have your liver enzymes checked every three months just to be safe.

5. Risk factors can predispose drug-induced myopathy, including being female, being an elderly patient, the duration of

therapy, high doses of statins, renal/liver dysfunction, a concurrent thyroid problem, decreased albumin levels, Lupus, vigorous or excessive duration of exercise, and known drug interactions (statins plus fibrates or nicotinic acid and statins in addition to cytochrome P450 3A4 inhibitors, which are liver enzymes that help rid the body of drugs and that certain drugs can affect).[64]

Lipid and Liver Monitoring Parameters

What It Is	Abbreviation	Normal Number
LIPID PANEL		
Total cholesterol	TC	<200 mg/dL
Bad cholesterol (low-density lipoprotein)	LDL	<130 mg/dL
Good cholesterol (high-density lipoprotein)	HDL	>40 mg/dL
Triglycerides	TG	<150 mg/dL
LIVER TESTS		
Liver enzyme	ALT (alanine transaminase)	7–53 IU/L
Liver enzyme	AST (aspartate aminotransferase)	11–47 IU/L

VIOLATION OF RULE #7: Know Your Medication's Monitoring Parameters

Had Kyle been vigilant with his monitoring parameters (by keeping track of his lipid and liver-enzyme levels as listed in the above table), he and his doctor would have noticed the increase in his liver enzymes and checked more closely to make sure Kyle wasn't experiencing muscle problems.

VIOLATION OF RULE #9: Be Aware of Drug Interactions

Kyle, his doctor, and his pharmacist should have recognized what was happening with the interaction between his simvastatin and gemfibrozil. If any of the three had done their homework, they would have realized that Kyle should not have been on a dose of simvastatin higher than 10 mg. Kyle is on a dose that is four times too high. After Kyle waits nearly three weeks to see his physician, he has already experienced serious muscle breakdown related to his two cholesterol medications. He has a SCr of 2.6 mg/dL and myoglobin in his urine: Both are signs of serious kidney trouble. Fortunately, Kyle asked his pharmacist about his symptoms and followed the good advice he was given, which was that he should see his doctor right away. Kyle acts just in time to prevent serious kidney damage. It is important to know the symptoms of muscle breakdown if you are on a statin or a fibrate. Signs and symptoms of myopathy and rhabdomyolysis commonly include unexplained muscle pain or fatigue, dark urine, and tiredness or weakness. To make sure your liver is okay with the statins, you should have your liver function checked before you start a statin, with any dose increase, and every three months. Also avoid using a combination statin–fibrate therapy if you are more than seventy years old, have liver or kidney impairment, have skeletal muscle dysfunction, are taking cyclosporine or tacrolimus, and have taken macrolides (erythromycin, azithromycin) or azole antifungal agents (clotrimazole, ketoconazole) for long periods of time.[65] If you are on a statin and gemfibrozil (Lopid) or Tricor, rhabdomyolysis is a real possibility. I am seeing this problem more and more frequently. Don't think this can't happen to you.

 VIOLATION OF RULE #16: Ads Don't Warn of Incidence of Adverse Events—Don't Believe Them

A recent Lipitor commercial stated that muscle pain and weakness are a sign of a rare but serious side effect and to contact your doctor if this occurs—but how rare is this event? The problem is that the drug manufacturer doesn't tell you. Information from other sources estimates the incidence of drug-induced rhabdomyolysis from statins occurs in anywhere from 0.1 to 7 percent of cases. If 55,122,000 people were on just Lipitor in 2007, then is this really a rare occurrence?[66] I think not. Billions of people take statins every day. Just to estimate, let's multiply one billion people by 0.1 percent. This comes out to one hundred million people who may experience this adverse event. Don't be one of them. Know your information before starting this drug.

Medication-Induced Hyperkalemia (High Blood Potassium Levels)

The following case shows us that some medications can cause hyperkalemia, a condition that indicates high levels of potassium in your blood.

THE PATIENT

Natalie is a sixty-four-year-old woman who is usually energetic and busy. She enjoys volunteering at the local Red Cross and baking pies for her grandchildren. She feels that the past two years have really taken a toll on her generally good health. Natalie's primary care physician diagnoses her with highly elevated blood pressure and starts her on two medications: spironolactone and ramipril. Her blood pressure has been difficult for her to control. Two months ago, she was in a car accident. She was not seriously injured, but since the accident she has experienced terrible neck pain.

THE SYMPTOMS

A few days ago, Natalie began to have trouble getting around. She says she feels like all the strength in her legs is gone. At first she writes off the inconvenience as just another symptom of getting older or maybe something lingering from the accident. After the weakness consistently becomes worse over a few weeks, she decides to seek professional help.

THE SUSPECTS

The likely suspects are the following drugs.

1. Ramipril (Trade Name: Altace)

Ramipril is used for high blood pressure. It is known to cause a cough (7–12 percent), low blood pressure (11 percent), headache (1–5 percent), and high potassium levels (1–10 percent). Ramipril is in the ever-popular class of antihypertensives known as angiotensin-converting enzyme (ACE) inhibitors. As with other ACE inhibitors, ramipril (Altace) is commonly prescribed and ranked forty-third among the top two hundred drugs prescribed in 2006.[67] A black box warning states that usage should be avoided in pregnancy. ACE inhibitors can cause injury and death to a developing fetus when used in the second and third trimesters. Patients should discontinue ACE inhibitors as soon as pregnancy is detected.[68]

2. Metaxalone (Trade Name: Skelaxin)

Metaxalone relaxes muscles and relieves pain. It can cause drowsiness, dizziness, anxiety, upset stomach, and irritability. It can also cause motion and reaction impairment. Be careful when taking this medication and working around machinery or driving. It is not recommended to take Metaxalone with alcohol or sedatives, such as diazepam (Valium). This combination may have additive effects.[69]

3. Spironolactone (Trade Name: Aldactone)

Spironolactone lowers blood pressure and increases low potassium, heart failure, liver cirrhosis, and certain types of steroid overproduction. It can cause diarrhea (up to 29 percent), erectile dysfunction, male breast enlargement (9 percent), menstrual irregularities, and hyperkalemia (2 percent). Spironolactone has antiandrogen (anti-testosterone steroid) actions, so it is used for treating baldness in men and excessive hair growth in women.[70]

LET'S RECAP

Patient: Natalie, age 64
1. Ramipril (Altace) for high blood pressure: 5 mg daily

2. Metaxalone (Skelaxin) for Muscle pain: 800 mg 3 times daily
3. Spironolactone (Aldactone) for high blood pressure: 25 mg daily
Lab-test results:
  Potassium (K): 7.4 mEq/L (normally 3.5−5.2 mEq/L)
  Sodium (Na): 139 mEq/L (normally 135−145 mEq/L)
  BUN (blood urea nitrogen): 25 mg/dL (normally 7−18 mg/dL)
  SCr (sodium creatinine): 1.9 mg/dL (normally 0.6−1.2 mg/dL)
Other tests: EKG: Peaked T-waves

SUMMARY REPORT

An initial evaluation of the situation suggests that Natalie's high blood pressure is not directly causing the symptoms and that the following information must be considered:

- Natalie's blood urea nitrogen (BUN) and sodium creatinine (SCr), measures of kidney function, are elevated, meaning she has slightly decreased kidney function.

- The EKG reveals the electrical pattern her heart produces is showing abnormalities.

- The potassium in her blood is highly elevated, which may cause the abnormalities on her EKG. The normal range is 3.5 to 5 mEq/L. Natalie's is way, way too high.

- The sodium level in her blood is normal.

SOLVE THE MYSTERY

From her symptoms and lab tests, we can develop a clearer picture of what is occurring. We can rule out metaxalone immediately, because it relieves pain and does not cause weakness. We now must look at the bad behaviors of the remaining two drugs. We can see that both drugs can cause hyperkalemia (high blood potassium). Looking at the lab-test results, we see that Natalie's blood potassium level is indeed elevated. After evaluating all the evidence, we can identify the guilty parties.[71]

The Culprit: Ramipril

Ramipril is a member of the ACE inhibitor class of drugs. Other

ACE inhibitors include lisinopril, enalapril and hydrochlorothiazide (Vaseretic), benazepril, moexipril, and fosinopril. These medications decrease the production of a substance called angiotensin that increases blood pressure. Angiotensin regulates many vasculature systems, including sodium and water retention in the kidneys. However, as a consequence, the body retains potassium, because it is usually exchanged for sodium. Normally this excess potassium is no big deal when no other drugs cause the same problem and nothing else is malfunctioning in the body. In Natalie's case, this is not the situation. Her blood tests show her kidney function is slightly decreased. The kidneys usually get rid of potassium if the body does not need it. However, her kidneys are not working well enough to keep up.[72]

The Accomplice: Spironolactone

The drug spironolactone is an aldosterone antagonist. Aldosterone is a hormone that increases blood pressure by allowing sodium and water to stay in the body. Spironolactone belongs to a class of diuretics known as potassium-sparing diuretics. This means that spironolactone does not allow enough potassium to leave the body and instead tries to keep as much potassium as possible from being excreted through the kidneys and urine. Being prescribed this medication, which increases potassium in the body, should have prompted Natalie to have her potassium levels checked. Too much potassium is responsible for the weak feeling in Natalie's legs.[73]

THE SOLUTION

Natalie's situation is urgent. Untreated hyperkalemia can cause an irregular heartbeat and can ultimately be fatal. The treatment consists of stabilizing the heart muscle with intravenous calcium. Doctors then use a potassium binder called Kayexalate to decrease the total amount of potassium in the body.

The long-term treatment is to replace the spironolactone Natalie is using with a medication that does not cause the same reaction. Natalie's spironolactone is replaced with another diuretic that actually promotes potassium loss, a medication called furosemide (Lasix). Natalie should have blood tests to check her kidney function along with her potassium and electrolytes about every three months to determine if everything is working as planned. If not, she has many other treatment options, such as triamterene or hydrochlorothiazide.

WHAT ARE YOUR CHANCES?

Hyperkalemia is seen regularly in the hospital, and an estimated 1 to 10 percent of patients present with hyperkalemia. However, this is another drug-induced problem that goes largely unreported to the FDA.[74] In 2007 there were seventeen reports of hyperkalemia associated with ramipril and sixteen reported cases of spironolactone-related incidents.[75] The consensus is that this problem has a low risk of occurrence if this type of drug is taken alone. When combined with another drug that causes potassium retention or kidney dysfunction, the chances of an adverse reaction are much higher. In fact, one source stated that the interaction is one of the top ten to look out for and to aggressively avoid. Altace (ramipril) had an estimated 6,036,000 prescriptions dispensed in 2006.[76] (6,036,000 Rxs/12 Rxs per patient-year = 503,000 patients × 1–10 percent = 5,030–50,300 cases of hyperkalemia/year.)

HELPFUL ADVICE

Hyperkalemia is common among patients on ACE inhibitors (such as lisinopril, ramipril, vaseretic [Enalapril], moexipril, or fosinopril), ARBs (such as losartan [Cozaar], Atacand [candesartan], Avalide [irbesartan], Diovan [valsartan], or Micardis [telmisartan]), and aldosterone antagonists. However, no specific data report the incidence of hyperkalemia while on ACE inhibitors and spironolactone. Some factors that predispose you to hyperkalemia that you and your physician should be aware of include reduced renal function (kidney function), diabetes, and advanced heart failure. Your physician should regularly check your blood for potassium levels to avoid a trip to the hospital. You should have your renal function (creatinine clearance [CrCl]) and serum electrolytes (potassium) checked every three months while on either spironolactone or an ACE inhibitor; however, most cases are asymptomatic and go unreported. In this case, Natalie should have followed Rules #2 and #6. Knowing her kidney lab values and having her potassium levels regularly screened could have prevented a hospitalization.

It is important to recognize the signs and symptoms of hyperkalemia, which most commonly include nausea, fatigue, muscle weakness, or tingling sensations. Serious symptoms include a slow heartbeat and a weak pulse. Your primary-care physician should monitor such factors as kidney function and potassium through regular blood tests. Always go to the lab to have these tests performed. Even though it may feel inconvenient if these evaluations always come back normal, one day these simple tests could keep you out of the hospital.[77]

Another way to avoid a trip to the hospital is to stop taking the next dose of your blood pressure medications (ACE inhibitors and ARBs) if you are sick and dehydrated, such as when you have the flu. These medications are just one class of drugs that can accumulate in your body if you are dehydrated and your kidney function is not optimal. Kidney specialists suggest taking a blood pressure reading, laying off the next dose of your medications if your blood pressure is not too high, and calling the doctor. Continuing to use your medication and failing to immediately contact your doctor will do much more harm than good, such as causing renal failure, particularly if you continue your medication upon the onset of symptoms, versus missing one dose of your meds.

 VIOLATION OF RULE #2: Know Your Kidney "Lab Values"

If Natalie and her physician had been vigilant in knowing her kidney lab values and Lab-Test Schedule, her hospitalization could have been prevented. The monitoring parameters for ramipril and spironolactone include checking renal function and electrolytes (potassium) before starting treatment and every three months thereafter.

VIOLATION OF RULE #6: Know Your Lab-Test Schedule

Some diseases, such as diabetes, reduced kidney function, and advanced heart failure, increase the risk for hyperkalemia. If you have these conditions, closely monitor your potassium level. Natalie and her doctor should have been checking this regularly. Natalie should also have recognized the signs and symptoms of hyperkalemia: muscle weakness, fatigue, nausea, and tingling sensations. Serious symptoms include a weak pulse or slow heartbeat. Many patients take spironolactone and an ACE inhibitor, such as ramipril. It is important to stick to your lab-monitoring schedule and to not miss those appointments.

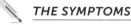 **CONDITION**

Medication-Induced Diarrhea

The following case shows us that some medications can cause life-threatening, contagious diarrhea.

 THE PATIENT

Jim is an eighty-three-year-old man from Illinois. He has farmed all his life and enjoys his slow-paced life. Jim was always in great health until two years ago, when he fell and broke his hip trying to get on his tractor. While undergoing rehabilitation, he was diagnosed with high cholesterol and high blood pressure. He was given medicines to treat these problems. Jim's farming days are now over, but he still tries to do what he can around the house. Recently, he was trying to clear the snow from his porch and came down with pneumonia. He goes to the doctor and is given an antibiotic and told to rest.

THE SYMPTOMS

A couple of days after Jim finishes his antibiotics, he is feeling better but not great. While watching television, he starts to have severe pain in his gut. Shortly after this, Jim begins having uncontrollable diarrhea. Nothing he takes for it works, and after a couple of days, he becomes dehydrated and has to go to the hospital.

THE SUSPECTS

The likely suspects are the following drugs.

1. Ezetimibe (Trade Name: Zetia)

Ezetimibe decreases cholesterol by decreasing the amount of cholesterol the body gets from food. It can also cause abdominal pain (3 percent), diarrhea (3–4 percent), headache (8 percent), joint pain (4 percent), and muscle pain (extremely rare). Ezetimibe is usually considered to have minimal side effects.[78]

2. Amoxicillin and Clavulanic Acid (Trade Name: Augmentin)

Amoxicillin and clavulanic acid are used as an antibiotic to help cure bacterial infections. They can cause nausea, vomiting, diarrhea, upset stomach, and skin rashes. Amoxicillin has also been found to cause serious allergic reactions that can be life-threatening. Always be aware of previous antibiotics taken that may have triggered similar reactions.

Additionally, amoxicillin and clavulanic acid, like many other antibiotics, can cause an inflammation of the bowels due to its nonspecific killing of many bacteria. This allows bad bacteria to start growing and can cause damage to the intestinal tract.[79]

3. Atenolol (Trade Name: Tenormin)

Atenolol is used for high blood pressure, heart problems, and chest pain (angina). The most common adverse effects are low blood pressure, dizziness, fatigue, and lethargy or weakness in 1 to 10 percent of patients.[80] Despite being a fairly old drug, atenolol ranked thirty-fourth of the top two hundred prescribed for 2006.[81] An approximation is that more than 1.5 million prescriptions of atenolol were dispensed in 2006.

LET'S RECAP

Patient: Jim, age 83

1. Ezetimibe (Zetia) for high cholesterol: 10 mg daily
2. Amoxicillin/clavulanic acid (Augmentin) for pneumonia:
   500/125 mg every 8 hours
3. Atenolol (Tenormin) for High blood pressure: 50 mg daily

Lab-test results:

　　Potassium (K): 3.4 mEq/L (normally 3.5–5.2 mEq/L)

　　Sodium (Na): 132 mEq/L (normally 135–145 mEq/L)

　　WBC (white blood cell count): 17,900 (normally 4,500–10,000)

　　Temp: 102°F (normally 98.6°F)

Other tests: *C. diff* assay: positive

SUMMARY REPORT

An initial evaluation of the situation suggests that Jim's high cholesterol levels and high blood pressure are not directly causing the symptoms and that the following information must be considered:

- Jim develops another fever even after the antibiotics cure his pneumonia.

- He has high numbers of white blood cells, which usually means he has some type of infection.

- Jim has been taking his other medications for a long time prior to this episode.

- His stool tests positive for a bacterium called *Clostridium difficile* (*C. diff*).

- Jim's sodium and potassium are slightly low, which may mean he has lost too much fluid from the diarrhea.

SOLVE THE MYSTERY

Jim has always been healthy and has lived an active lifestyle until recently. From the information given on his medications, atenolol can be eliminated immediately as the likely suspect. Jim has been taking ezetimibe for about two years, and this problem would have arisen earlier if that drug were the culprit. It then becomes obvious which medication is causing his problems.

The Culprits: Amoxicillin and Clavulanic Acid

This antibiotic combination is notorious for causing diarrhea. Amoxicillin itself is known to cause this condition as well, but in combination with clavulanic acid, the rate goes way up. Clavulanic acid is not an antibiotic itself; however, it helps protect amoxicillin from bacteria. Bacteria can release specialized proteins that break down amoxicillin, but clavulanic acid blocks this reaction from happening. Therefore, this combination can cure a broader spectrum of bacteria, which can be good and bad. It is good when the antibiotic helps patients and their infections are cured. It is bad when the combination kills all the good bacteria in the intestines and allows the bad bacteria to grow and to overpopulate. The bad bacteria in Jim's case, a bug called *C. diff*, cannot be killed by amoxicillin alone or with clavulanic acid. These bacteria grow fast with no competition from the good bacteria that have all been killed. *C. diff* bacteria can release toxins that damage the intestines and cause the pain and severe diarrhea that Jim experiences.[82]

THE SOLUTION

This type of diarrhea is treated with further antibiotic therapy; however, the antibiotics target the bad bacteria that have taken over his intestines.[83] Jim is given metronidazole 500 mg three times daily for ten to fourteen days.[84] Any antidiarrheal medication Jim is on has to be stopped, because it may increase the severity of his condition. An essential part of Jim's therapy is to maintain good hygiene with proper hand washing. *C. diff* is easily spread from close contact with infected patients.

WHAT ARE YOUR CHANCES?

Seven percent of all adverse drug events are due to drug-induced diarrhea, and more than seven hundred drugs are to blame, with 25 percent of them being antibiotics.[85] In the United States, an estimated three million cases of *Clostridium difficile*–associated diarrhea (CDAD) and colitis occur each year. Several risk factors may predispose you to *C. diff* colitis, such as advanced age (>60), hospitalization, and exposure to antibiotics (clindamycins, cephalosporins, and penicillins).[86] *C. diff* causes 10 to 20 percent of antibiotic-associated diarrhea. Most of these cases occur in the hospital. About 10 percent of patients in the hospital for more than two days develop CDAD. This can occur while the patient is still in the hospital or a few days thereafter. The number of cases of CDAD is actually increasing. This increase has many reasons, most notably larger populations of nursing home residents and larger numbers of antibiotics being prescribed. Outside a hospital or nursing home, it is less common, affecting about 1 to 3 people per 100,000.[87] The key risk factor for the development is antibiotic use. Clindamycin has the largest association with CDAD. High occurrences also link penicillins (such as amoxicillin or ampicillin) and cephalosporins (such as Rocephin, Omnicef, or cephalexin) as accomplices. The incidence of antibiotic-associated diarrhea in patients who are taking amoxicillin/clavulanate nears 10 to 15 percent. Let's take a look at the incidence of diarrhea with other antibiotics: clindamycin (2–20 percent); macrolides, such as azithromycin and erythromycin (>10 percent); penicillins, such as amoxicillin and ampicillin (1–20 percent); quinolones, such as ciprofloxacin and levofloxacin (2 percent); sulfonamides (1–2 percent); and tetracyclines (1–10 percent).[88] In 2007 the FDA's MedWatch system reported two cases of *C. diff* colitis induced by Augmentin (amoxicillin and clavulanic acid).[89] This number is a far cry from the total number of cases of colitis that the combination of amoxicillin and clavulanic acid has caused.

HELPFUL ADVICE

C. diff colitis is common among hospitalized and nursing home patients. It does occur among the general population, but at a much lower rate. If you develop diarrhea after taking a course of antibiotics, talk with your doctor if the symptoms are severe and involve cramping and dehydration. If you do have CDAD, it will change the way in which treatment proceeds. In this case, following Rule #8 may have helped Jim. Taking something for his diarrhea was not a good idea here.[90]

Always contact a physician if diarrhea persists longer than one to two days. After this time period, many other problems can develop as a result of the loss of water and electrolytes (sodium, potassium, and chloride). Tell a health-care professional if you were on a recent course of antibiotics. The best prevention is to use antibiotics only when completely necessary. Avoid going to a physician to request antibiotics; chances are you do not need them to get over an illness. Contact a physician immediately if you experience extreme tiredness, fainting, or bloody stools.[91]

Prevent diarrhea by maintaining proper fluid intake and diet; avoiding artificial sweeteners; using antibiotics only when necessary and reserving broad spectrum antibiotics for serious illness; adjusting doses to fit age, weight, renal/hepatic function; taking drugs with meals if allowed; eating frequent small meals; using drugs with a low risk of diarrhea when possible; and avoiding liquid medications with a high sorbitol content.[92]

Hygiene is the best way to combat *C. diff* colitis. Washing your hands often is the easiest way to prevent spread and transmission; in the hospital, this is extremely important, because your chances of getting *C. diff* while in the hospital are much greater. This recommendation extends to your family and nursing staff. Spores spread *C. diff* from the fecal to oral route. The spores can stay active for a very long time, so it is important to wash all bed sheets, clothing, and handrails thoroughly.

 VIOLATION OF RULE #8: Do Not Hesitate to Call Your Doctor

Had Jim contacted his doctor sooner, his physician may have recognized this diarrhea as a more serious problem. Jim is unlucky with his prescribed antibiotic. When at home, patients are much less likely to contract *C. diff* colitis; however, this does not remove the risk completely. If diarrhea persists for more than one to two days, contact your doctor, and remind him or her about your recent antibiotic use. It is also important to remember that C. *diff* colitis can appear weeks after the antibiotic therapy is over. Hygiene is the best weapon against contracting C. *diff*. Frequent hand washing with antimicrobial soap is important. Medications can treat the infection once it is confirmed to be C. *diff*. If you are experiencing diarrhea with antibiotics, remember to stay hydrated. Pedialyte is a great replacement for the fluids lost to diarrhea.

██████ CONDITION ██████

Medication-Induced Movement Disorder

The following case shows us that some medications can cause movement disorders that cause a person to move or shake uncontrollably, a situation that can be quite frightening.

THE PATIENT

Harry is a seventy-four-year-old man who feels he is in the prime of his life. He finally retired a few years back after starting his own company in 1965. He has moved out of the big city to a farm where he gets all the exercise he needs. The change in scenery has really lifted his spirits, and his stress has vanished. Harry's only health problems are his old war wound, heartburn, and the occasional cold. Things can't get much better for Harry.

THE SYMPTOMS

A few weeks back, Harry started to notice his left arm was shaking. He thinks at first that maybe he has had too much coffee. Then, his wife tells him to stop shaking his arm at dinner when he has no idea he is doing it. He begins to feel a little nauseated as well. His condition starts to concern him, so he goes to the local doctor for the first time. The doctor gives him a prescription for prochlorperazine (Compazine) for the nausea, which seems to make the shaking worse. After this happens, he decides to go to the emergency room.

THE SUSPECTS

The likely suspects are the following drugs.

1. Metoclopramide (Trade Name: Reglan)

Metoclopramide relieves heartburn symptoms and nausea/vomiting, and it treats static bowel disorders. It may cause drowsiness (10–70 percent), fatigue (~10 percent), muscle spasms/dyskinesias (uncontrolled movements in ~20 percent), and restlessness (~10 percent). Metoclopramide promotes upper-bowel movement, which largely accounts for its use, and also blocks transmitters in the brain from causing nausea and vomiting.[93]

2. Alprazolam (Trade Name: Xanax)

Alprazolam decreases anxiety and treats panic and seizure disorders. Side effects include drowsiness and sedation (>10 percent), fatigue (>10 percent), increased/decreased appetite (>10 percent), impaired coordination (>10 percent), and dry mouth (>10 percent).

Alprazolam is a controlled substance and has abuse potential. Because of possible overdose, patients should be monitored for lung and heart function closely. Withdrawal symptoms have been known to occur with patients on long-term therapy. Abruptly stopping treatment is not recommended. Alprazolam is not recommended for patients with narrow-angle glaucoma.[94]

3. Prochlorperazine (Trade Name: Compazine)

Proclorperazine relieves nausea and balance/coordination problems. It has been known to cause drowsiness, skin rashes, difficult-to-regulate blood sugar, decreased sex drive, male breast enlargement, difficulty urinating, movement disorders, Parkinsonism, and blurred vision. Prochlorperazine is related to antipsychotic medications and can be used for that purpose in some cases. It works by blocking transmitters in the brain that are responsible for nausea and vomiting.[95]

LET'S RECAP

Patient: Harry, age 74
1. Metoclopramide (Reglan) for heartburn: 5 mg daily
2. Alprazolam (Xanax) for anxiety: 0.5 mg 3 times daily
3. Prochlorperazine (Compazine) for nausea: 15 mg every 6–8 hours, as needed
Lab-test results: All within normal range
Other tests: Not applicable

SUMMARY REPORT

An initial evaluation of the situation suggests that no particular disease is causing the symptoms and that the following information must be considered:

- Harry's lab tests come back normal.

- His new doctor gives him a prescription for prochlorperazine (Compazine), and the shaking seems to worsen.

- Harry rarely takes his alprazolam anymore due to his laidback country lifestyle.

SOLVE THE MYSTERY

It looks like we have another problem that is missed initially. Harry goes in for a tremor in his arm and comes out worse off. Looking at his drug profile shows us a few interesting facts. First, we look at alprazolam. It does not appear to be the culprit here. Harry has gradually taken less after his move and stress reduction, so it is unlikely his reaction is occurring now. The shaking becomes worse after he is given prochlorperazine, so it seems to be involved somewhere. The most suspicious character looks to be metoclopramide, which is at the scene of the crime the entire time and has a terrible alibi.

The Culprit: Metoclopramide

The problem is metoclopramide the entire time. Harry has been taking this medication for a long time without problems. However, long-time use does not eliminate the chances of a patient's experiencing an adverse reaction. His recent lifestyle slow down may be allowing him to become more aware of his health problems. Regardless, metoclopramide can cause movement problems that are mainly due to the drug's dopamine-blocking properties. A reduction in dopamine is responsible for the movement problems seen in Parkinson's disease. Dopamine is responsible for maintaining the balance of movement in the intestines. Metoclopramide works by blocking the dopamine receptors in the brain, thereby reducing nausea and increasing movement in the GI (gastrointestinal) tract. However, the rest of the body relies on this dopamine to maintain its muscle coordination. When too many of the dopamine receptors are blocked, a drug-induced Parkinson's disease and similar symptoms begin to emerge. Therefore, the problem is in his brain, not in his hands.[96]

 ### The Accomplice: Prochlorperazine

Metoclopramide is not alone in this crime. Its assistant is prochlorperazine. Prochlorperazine has similar dopamine-blocking actions in the brain. Combining these two medications can have additive effects, as is evident in Harry's case. Luckily, Harry seeks medical attention. Even though his first doctor does not see the drug-induced problem, he does aid in the diagnosis by giving Harry prochlorperazine. The symptoms of this drug-induced problem can become worse and even irreversible over time. This rarely occurs with these two drugs but is common with drugs in the same class.[97]

 ### THE SOLUTION

Harry discontinues the prochlorperazine, and his doctor prescribes another drug for his heartburn instead of metoclopramide. The main problem in Harry's case is his formerly busy lifestyle. He had no time for doctors then, so he always insisted on refills of his old medications. However, many new drugs have emerged for the treatment of his condition that have fewer side effects and are more effective. His new medication for heartburn is Prilosec, which is available over the counter. The tremors will most likely never affect him again.

WHAT ARE YOUR CHANCES?

One source stated that patients taking metoclopramide were at a fourfold increased risk for movement disorders when compared with patients not taking metoclopramide.[98] Metoclopramide-induced movement disorders occur in an estimated <1 to 25 percent of individuals taking the medication. One in five hundred patients may experience these symptoms while on the usual doses of 30 to 40 mg/day, and reactions are usually seen within the first twenty-four to forty-eight hours of treatment. Pediatric patients, adults younger than thirty, and patients who are on higher doses due to treatment of cancer-related nausea are at a higher risk of these movement disorders.[99] However, most of these reactions are minor. These effects are highly dose- and age-related. (6,325,000 Rxs/12 Rxs per patient-year = 527,083 patients × 1–25 percent = 5,271–131,770 cases of movement disorders.) In 2007 fifty-two cases of movement disorders were reported to the FDA's MedWatch site.[100]

HELPFUL ADVICE

A movement disorder can be a common reaction if certain drugs are taken in combination. However, with the wide range of reported incidence, it is unclear just how common this complication actually is. If you have unexplained movements while on metoclopramide, contact your doctor immediately. Harry's situation is an example of not following Rule #11. Harry eventually goes to the ER, but he should have been more aware of his condition sooner. He also does not follow Rule #15. His prochlorperazine dose is too high as well. This medication should be used at 5 to 10 mg three to four times a day, with a maximum dose of 40 mg a day. Prochlorperazine has a tendency to cause movement disorders and should only be used as a last resort in the management of behavioral problems in elderly patients. Also, due to its side effects, this is not a preferred drug for the prevention of nausea and vomiting in elderly patients.[101]

Much toxicity is age-related, as in Harry's case, and may emerge after years of treatment. Some risk factors are advanced age, cognitive impairment, being female, iron deficiency, mental retardation, rapid dose escalation, or high doses of antipsychotics.[102] Movement disorders can be manifested as involuntary movements of the arms and legs, restlessness, facial grimacing, sticking out the tongue continuously, lip smacking, difficulty breathing and swallowing, rigidity, stooped posture, turning the head, and symptoms resembling tetanus (clenching and weakness).[103] Parkinson's-like symptoms may show up within six months and can subside after two to three months of discontinuing the drug. Be on the lookout for these symptoms, and if they occur, stop taking your medication and see your doctor immediately.[104] Some of these adverse effects can be severe and irreversible. It is important to remember that if you notice something that isn't right, you need to contact your doctor or pharmacist immediately. Movement problems are a prime example of something that doesn't happen suddenly. Harry notices this change and goes to his doctor. Be sure to do the same.

 VIOLATION OF RULE #11: If Your Health Changes after You Add a New Drug, Think Drug-Induced Disease

Everything is fine for Harry until a new medication is added that makes him aware of his problem. Harry may have had problems with movement before, but he was either too busy to notice or it took adding one more medication to cause him to recognize his movement problems. Fortunately, with his wife's observance, Harry contacts his doctor. Some movement problems due to medications can be serious and irreversible if not caught early.

VIOLATION OF RULE #15: Remember That Elderly Individuals Should Be on Lower Doses

If you notice any shakiness, uncontrollable movement, trouble walking, or difficulty moving, contact your doctor to set up an appointment. A medication that you are taking could cause your symptoms. Some of the common offenders include conventional antipsychotic medications (such as haloperidol, chlorpromazine, thioridazine, or perphenazine), nausea medications (prochlorperazine, droperidol, promethazine, metoclopramide), SSRIs (such as sertraline or paroxetine), tricyclic antidepressants (such as amitriptyline, clomipramine, or doxepine), antiepileptics (phenytoin, carbamazepine, valproate), levodopa, and pimozide.[105]

To prevent this problem from occurring, use the lowest effective dose, because high doses of these medications can lead to movement disorders, orthostatic hypotension (dizziness when you stand or sit up due to changes in blood pressure), sleepiness, and anticholinergic effects (such as loss of coordination, confusion, increased heart rate, shaking, decreased bowel movements and urination, or pupil dilation).[106] Slowly increasing doses of medications with the potential to cause movement disorders and using atypical antipsychotics instead of conventional antipsychotics are another way to help prevent these complications. Using a short course of antimuscarinic agents (benztropine, diphenhydramine, trihexyphenidyl) during the first weeks of treatment for movement issues has proven to be effective in younger patients receiving high-potency antipsychotics.[107] These medications are not considered first-line medications for the elderly due to the risk of side effects. If you are on one of these drugs, look for alternatives. Use the medication only when needed and not for an excessive amount of time. In this case, Harry may have been able to solve his nausea if he were able to control his heartburn with a different medication, such as a proton pump inhibitor (such as omeprazole, pantoprazole, or lansoprazole).

Medication-Induced Problems from Lack of Oversight

The following case clearly indicates the importance of patients asking medical professionals to exert oversight and go through the process of medication reconciliation to prevent adverse drug reactions. It also points out that patients need to keep their own accurate and complete drug list no matter where they are within the health-care system. (A blank form for creating this list is included in the Appendix.) The following case also shows us that medication lists constantly need to be reconciled. Reconciliation is a process in which a patient's medication list is kept accurate through the admission and discharge process of hospitals and other medical facilities.

THE PATIENT

Darlene is a seventy-seven-year-old recent widow. She enjoys knitting for her daughter who lives in town and also enjoys window watching to pass the day. Darlene is a naturally "nervous" lady who likes things neat. She currently takes a medication called clonazepam to control her anxiety attacks. Lately, she has been dealing with some hard times. Her husband passed away about a year ago, and today she is taken to the hospital due to an automobile accident on her way to a craft store. After Darlene has surgery, the physician decides to add diazepam to her drug regimen to relax her muscles. A few days later, she is released from the hospital and is told to continue to take the medications that her doctor has prescribed.

THE SYMPTOMS

A few days after she leaves the hospital, Darlene tries to go about her normal activities, but she finds it difficult to get around. She continues to take her routine drugs and the medications that her doctor has recently prescribed. One day Darlene's daughter comes over to eat lunch and notices that Darlene is acting very unusually.

She is telling Charlie to sit, but Charlie was her dog that passed away ten years ago. Darlene tells her daughter that she feels very dizzy and cannot see very well.

Darlene says she feels drunk, yet she knows she hasn't had any alcohol. When she gets up to "pet" Charlie, she falls. Luckily, her daughter is there and calls for help. Darlene is taken to the hospital with a broken arm and a diagnosis of change in mental status. While there, she also receives supportive care until the doctor figures out what has happened.

THE SUSPECTS

The likely suspects are the following drugs.

1. Acetaminophen (Trade Name: Tylenol)

Acetaminophen is used for a variety of problems, including dysmenorrhea (pain during menstruation), fever, headache, mild to moderate pain, postoperative pain, and osteoporosis. It can cause rash, GI bleed, and liver and kidney toxicity. Patients should not drink alcohol while on this medication or take more than 4,000 mg a day, because doing so can cause serious liver damage. Patients should also watch for signs of bleeding while on this medication.[108]

2. Clonazepam (Trade Name: Klonopin)

Clonazepam is usually used to treat anxiety but may also be used for seizure disorders, restless leg syndrome, and sleepwalking. Some side effects include ataxia (loss of muscle coordination; seen in 30 percent of seizure disorder patients and 5 percent in panic disorder patients), behavior problems (50 percent in seizure disorders), dizziness, impaired cognition, seizure, aggravation, somnolence (drowsiness; 37 percent in panic disorders), respiratory depression (decreased ability of the body to get oxygen), paradoxical reactions (the opposite of what is expected), slurred speech, blurred vision, and a glassy-eyed appearance. Clonazepam is in the class of medications known as the benzodiazepines, which may be addictive. It is a controlled substance.[109]

3. Diazepam (Trade Name: Valium)

Diazepam is often used for anxiety but can be used for a number of purposes, such as treatment of alcohol withdrawal, skeletal muscle relaxer, relief of seizure disorders, sedation, and as a muscle relaxer. It can cause hypotension (low blood pressure), ataxia, drowsiness, respiratory depression, slurred speech, nausea and vomiting, seizures, dizziness, headaches, tremor, and blurred vision. Diazepam is also a benzodiazepine.[110]

LET'S RECAP

Patient: Darlene, age 77
1. Acetaminophen (Tylenol) for pain from postsurgery: 1,000 mg every 6 hours, as needed
2. Clonazepam (Klonopin) for panic disorder: 1 mg 3 times daily, as needed
3. Diazepam (Valium) as a muscle relaxer: 1 mg every 8 hours
Lab-test results:
　Benzodiazepines: (+) positive
Other tests: Broken left arm

SUMMARY REPORT

An initial evaluation of the situation suggests that a disease is not causing the symptoms and the following information must be considered:

- Darlene was already on two medications prior to her accident.
- Darlene is on two medications that can alter mental status. She falls due to dizziness.

SOLVE THE MYSTERY

Darlene's physician decides to run a drug screen and notices a high level of benzodiazepines in her system. He then realizes that maybe she has some other medications at home. Sure enough, he calls the pharmacy she uses regularly and sees that she is on both diazepam and clonazepam.

The Culprits: Clonazepam and Diazepam

Darlene's problem occurs because the prescription for diazepam is a standing order given after surgery to help relax Darlene's muscles. A standing order consists of preprinted forms that doctors use to cover all possible contingencies so they are not bothered in the middle of the night. They don't always look to see whether the patient is already on a similar medication or if the new medication interferes with the patient's current regimen. In other words, they do not engage in the process of medication reconciliation (explained in Chapter 1 and also discussed later in the "Helpful Advice" section of this case). Darlene is released from the hospital with both her home medication, clonazepam (Klonopin), *and* with the medication she took while hospitalized, diazepam. The problem is that clonazepam and diazepam are benzodiazepines, and their effects are additive. The end result is that Darlene becomes toxic due to being prescribed two different drugs from the same class. Taking too many benzodiazepines can cause an overabundance of side effects, such as respiratory depression, confusion, dizziness, blurred vision, and sleepiness. As in Darlene's situation, these can lead to someone's feeling drunk or even experiencing a fall. Also, side effects of these medications can be seen especially in elderly patients, because their renal function may be decreased, which means more of the drug stays in their bodies because it can't be removed in the urine. The true danger in this situation is that Darlene is on clonazepam, and this is a drug that should not be used with elderly patients.

Benzodiazepines may account for up to 10 percent of drug-associated hospital admissions, and use among elderly patients has been associated with intellectual and cognitive impairment (abnormal changes in the brain, such as problems with language, reasoning, and judgment).[111] As Rule #4 states, elderly patients are different from younger people because of changes that occur in their bodies as they age. Benzodiazepines are listed on the *Beers Criteria for Potentially Inappropriate Medication Use in the Elderly*. The 2003 updated version of this list can be found at http://www.dcri.duke

.edu/ccge/curtis/beers.html.[112] This website lists medications that elderly patients should generally avoid unless it is absolutely necessary because they may pose more of a risk than a benefit.

Patients should use the lowest dose possible and increase the dose slowly if they must be on one of these drugs. Elderly individuals should be on lower doses of medications anyway, because their bodies do not eliminate medications as efficiently as those of younger individuals (due to decreased liver or kidney function).

THE SOLUTION

While in the hospital, Darlene is given fluids and oxygen to raise her oxygen levels and blood pressure. She is also given flumazenil (Romazicon), which is a benzodiazepine antagonist, meaning it reverses the effects of benzodiazepines, such as diazepam and clonazepam. A cast is placed on her broken arm. The doctor decides to discontinue the diazepam. Darlene is also cautioned about the use of benzodiazepines and pain medications. She vows to be more aware of her medications the next time.

WHAT ARE YOUR CHANCES?

In 2005 a total of 67,593 benzodiazepine ingestions were reported to U.S. poison control centers. These 67,593 ingestions included 3,018 major toxicities and 243 deaths. From 1995 to 2002 the occurrence of emergency department visits involving benzodiazepines increased by 41 percent.[113] A search of the FDA's MedWatch reports during three quarters of 2007 revealed three falls, one mental status change, and eleven overdoses for patients on diazepam. For patients on clonazepam, one case of delirium, three cases of dizziness, and one overdose were reported.[114] This report shows that the side effects of this medication are not being recorded. Also, not only are the two drugs causing side effects, but the major overall problem is the ineffective use of medication reconciliation. Multiple organizations have shown that medication reconciliation accounts for 46 percent of all medication errors at transition points (admissions, transfers, and discharges) and 20 percent of adverse events in hospitalized patients.[115] This is why it is important for you to read this book and learn what symptoms and reactions to watch for. These drugs are very popular. In 2006 there were 18,152,000 prescriptions a year for clonazepam and 12,764,000 prescriptions for diazepam.[116] In Darlene's case, due to improper medication reconciliation, the use of diazepam and clonazepam leads to a major drug interaction that results in excessive CNS effects, such as drowsiness, dizziness, and imbalance. In elderly patients, benzodiazepines should be avoided.

HELPFUL ADVICE

This case shows the importance of medication reconciliation, the act of obtaining the most accurate list of possible medications that the patient is currently on and comparing it with the doctor's list of medications at each transition, including the drug name, dosage, frequency, and route. This procedure makes sure that you are taking the medications that you should and are not taking any medications that are contraindicated. One study showed that implementing a program to help ensure this practice could decrease the rate of medication errors by 70 percent and reduce adverse drug events by more than 15 percent.[117] When medication was reconciled, the opportunities for drug interactions and duplications of medications were minimized, as in Darlene's case. She is prescribed diazepam, which is in the same class of medications that she is already on, and the doctor doesn't know she is taking clonazepam. Too much of this medication in her system causes toxic side effects.

In 2005 The Joint Commission set a National Patient Safety Goal to include medication reconciliation. In 2006 Joint Commission–accredited hospitals achieved a national average performance of 66.1 percent in developing a process to ensure that reconciliation occurred and 72.5 percent in communicating this information with the next care provider. The goal only had a 54 percent compliance rate. This information proves that the adherence rates are not adequate, so you need to be proactive in making sure you are safe.[118]

You play a very important role in making sure this medication reconciliation process occurs. Make a list of all your medications and present it to your doctor each time you visit. Include the names of all of your OTC medications and herbals, dosages, times, and how you take them. (A blank form for recording this information ["My Medicine Record"]can be found in the Appendix.) If your doctor or nurse adds, changes, or stops a medication, update your list. If possible, obtain a copy of your medical records once you leave the hospital and give a copy to your pharmacist. Always ask the doctor which medications they want you to continue to take when you leave the hospital, and make sure your labs are available to your pharmacist so they can adjust your medications depending on how well your liver or kidneys are functioning. Also, ask your pharmacist to review your list to see whether the drugstore's list matches up to yours and to make sure that no drug interactions or duplications of medications occur. In case of an emergency, let your family members know where you keep this list so they will be able to bring it to the hospital. Don't expect that these reactions won't happen to you when you go home. The system is faulty, and this happens all the time. The Joint Commission is working to promote medication reconciliation and has developed guidelines on how to improve procedures in this area.

 VIOLATION OF RULE #13: Insist on Medication Reconciliation

All patients need to take some responsibility for their own health. One easy way to protect yourself is to provide an accurate medication list to your doctor and update the information on your list every time it changes. This type of record keeping significantly decreases the number of problems that can arise. The next step is to ask the medical professionals you interact with—doctors, nurses, pharmacists, and anyone else in the health-care system—to always compare your list of meds to their lists or to orders for new prescriptions. They then need to reconcile, or adjust, any duplicate, overlapping, or contraindicated medications on those lists and make sure that you are not given drugs that can harm your health. By keeping your medication list current and insisting on medication reconciliation, you will be taking steps that should help you avoid a high percentage of adverse drug events and medication errors.

VIOLATION OF RULE #15: Remember That Elderly Individuals Should Be on Lower Doses

Elderly individuals are also prone to more side effects, especially when taking benzodiazepines. The nursing guidelines recommend a maximum dose of 1.5 mg a day of clonazepam to be used for anxiety.[119] Also, diazepam is not recommended due to its long-acting activity. Long-acting benzodiazepines have been associated with falls in elderly patients. The Health Care Financing Administration discourages the use of this drug in patients in long-term-care facilities.[120] If you are on a benzodiazepine, be aware of what dose is safe for you. This is a big problem; the guidelines to help protect bad things from happening to patients exist for a reason.

CONDITION

Opiate Withdrawal

The following case shows us that when one is taken off of an opiate medication, such as morphine, codeine, and oxycontin, a withdrawal frequently occurs.

THE PATIENT

Wilmer is a sixty-seven-year-old man who is newly retired. He was a construction worker who always enjoyed the outdoors. He now spends his days out on his lake fishing for bass when he is not in pain. He is healthy for his age, but, as a result of his construction days, he experiences a significant amount of pain in his back. A construction accident years ago landed him in the hospital and subsequently led to multiple surgeries to correct his back problems. Now the aches are pretty constant. Wilmer uses hydrocodone/acetaminophen

(Lortab) and fentanyl patches to control this pain, and he also takes butorphanol (Stadol) nasal spray to help manage his migraines.

One day Wilmer is feeling good, so he takes off the fentanyl patch and decides to spend the day fishing. After he catches a few bass, he begins to feel a migraine coming on, so he decides to pack up his things and go home. At his house, he puts his fish away and takes his butorphanol (Stadol) nasally for the migraine. Then Wilmer lies down to rest and to let the migraine wear off.

THE SYMPTOMS

After a few hours, he suddenly feels like he is coming down with the flu. Wilmer is shaky, anxious, throwing up, sweaty, experiencing stomach pain, and just achy all over. He feels so horrible that he decides to call the doctor to determine what is wrong.

THE SUSPECTS

The likely suspects are the following drugs.

1. Fentanyl Patches (Trade Name: Duragesic)

Fentanyl patches are used for the management of chronic moderate to severe pain in people who are used to having high amounts of opioids. Some of the side effects of this medication are itching, fever (35 percent), sweating, constipation, nausea (24 percent) and vomiting (33 percent), confusion, dizziness, sedation (sleepiness), apnea (interruption in breathing; 3–10 percent), and hypoventilation and respiratory depression (slow and shallow breathing). Fentanyl patches are controlled substances and have a high abuse potential. Patients should not abruptly stop using the patches, because withdrawal symptoms may ensue.[121]

2. Hydrocodone and Acetaminophen (Trade Names: Lortab, Vicodin, Norco)

Hydrocodone and acetaminophen are used to relieve moderate to severe pain. They can cause nausea and vomiting, constipation, rashes, respiratory depression, and drowsiness. Hydrocodone is a controlled substance with a high abuse potential. Patients should not abruptly stop taking this medication, because withdrawal may occur. This medication includes acetaminophen, which can cause liver toxicities. A maximum daily dose of acetaminophen is 4,000 mg. Patients should talk with their pharmacist to make sure that none of the medications they are taking contain acetaminophen.[122]

3. Butorphanol (Trade Name: Stadol NS)

Butorphanol is used for the treatment of pain, migraines, anesthesia, labor pain, and opioid adverse reactions, such as itching. It can cause nausea and vomiting (13 percent), dizziness (19 percent), weakness (3–9 percent), drowsiness (30–40 percent), nasal congestion (13 percent), and withdrawal symptoms (<1 percent in clinical trials).[123] Butorphanol (Stadol) is a controlled substance that should be used with caution in patients who chronically take opioids. This medication works to stimulate and to block opioid receptors. When used by itself, butorphanol can control pain adequately, but when used with another opioid medication, it can block the effects and cause opioid withdrawal symptoms.

LET'S RECAP

Patient: Wilmer, age 67
1. Fentanyl patches (Duragesic) 25 mcg/hr every 72 hours
2. Hydrocodone/acetaminophen (Lortab, Norco, Vicodin) for chronic back pain: One 10/500 mg* tablet every 4 hours, as needed
3. Butorphanol (Stadol NS) for migraines: 1 mg followed by second dose in 1 hour, as needed
Lab-test results: Not applicable
Other tests: Dilated pupils

---

* This is the appropriate way to express the dosage for this combination drug. It reflects the concentrations of hydrocodone and acetaminophen each in the medication.

SUMMARY REPORT

An initial evaluation of the situation suggests that Wilmer's health conditions are not directly causing the symptoms and that the following information must be considered:

- Two offenders are causing the problem.

- Wilmer is experiencing withdrawal syndrome, which mimics the flu, with symptoms of restlessness, sweating, muscle spasms, pains, chills, stomach cramps, hot and cold flashes, nausea, vomiting, diarrhea, fast breathing, and heart irregularities.

SOLVE THE MYSTERY

Wilmer is experiencing opioid withdrawal. Let's look at our three suspects. Wilmer has been on two medications (fentanyl patches and Lortab and acetaminophen) previously. Fentanyl patches are discontinued at the time of the incident, so do they play a part? The hydrocodone and acetaminophen are there all along, so they may not have any part in this crime. Butorphanol is taken right when the problems start occurring. Can you solve this one?

The Culprits: Fentanyl Patches and Butorphanol

Fentanyl patches are known to cause withdrawal in patients who abruptly discontinue this medication. These patches are powerful opioids, and the medication alone can cause the symptoms that Wilmer is now experiencing. When butorphanol is added to his drug regimen, it just enhances the effect. Butorphanol stimulates opioid receptors to allow pain relief, but it also blocks some opioid receptors as well. Blocking opioid receptors in a patient who has been on long-term opioid therapy can cause a person to go into withdrawal. The combination of these two medications just enhances the withdrawal syndrome that Wilmer is experiencing.

THE SOLUTION

Had Wilmer realized the importance of not abruptly stopping his medications or had he known a little more about his medications, he may have saved himself some trouble and a trip to the hospital. Gradually tapering off the patches may have helped Wilmer, as well as avoiding butorphanol as a pain medication option. Wilmer is treated by adding clonidine and dicyclomine to help manage his symptoms.

WHAT ARE YOUR CHANCES?

In the FDA's MedWatch reports of three quarters in 2007, ten withdrawal syndromes with fentanyl and none with butorphanol were reported.[124] Another study showed withdrawal symptoms in 3.5 percent (283) of adverse reactions on butorphanol out of a total 8,114 adverse-effect reports.[125] (3,818,000 Rxs/12 Rxs per patient-year = 318,167 patients × 3.5 percent = 11,136 patients experiencing withdrawal symptoms on butorphanol.)[126] In 2003 $49,260,000 was spent in butorphanol sales, and it was rated number 140 in the top 200 generic drugs by retail sales.[127] Approximately 4,524,000 fentanyl prescriptions were written for patients in 2007. This is a large number of people who are opioid-tolerant and who can easily experience withdrawal symptoms from a such drug as butorphanol.[128]

HELPFUL ADVICE

Most of the time when patients are taking pain medications as prescribed, they have no problem with withdrawal symptoms. Problems can arise when a drug interaction occurs and if patients decide to abruptly stop their medications due to side effects or for financial reasons. Opioids are strong pain medications that your body can become addicted to over time. When taken away suddenly, your body will go into withdrawal. When you add a drug that has reversal effects on opioids, the withdrawal can become very severe. This is why it is important for you to know what your medications are treating. Wilmer also should have followed Rules #9 and #14 to avoid this unfortunate mishap.

When you are instructed to discontinue any medication that you have been on for a while, talk to your doctor or pharmacist to determine whether the medication you are on can be stopped or needs to be tapered off, such as with opioids. If you have been on a narcotic for more than a week, do not stop taking it suddenly, because it can throw you right into withdrawal. These medications need to be gradually decreased over time by first eliminating the "as-needed doses" and changing to "an average daily dose" (for example, every four to six hours). The Veterans Health Administration Clinical Practice Guidelines suggest regimens for tapering off opioids. These are just general guidelines, and tapering should be individualized for each patient. The tapering regimen for short-acting opioids is as follows: Decrease dose by 10 percent every 3 to 7 days, or reduce dose by 20 to 50 percent a day until lowest dosage form is reached. Then increase the dosing interval, eliminating one dose every 2 to 5 days. To decrease the dosing regimen for long-acting agents, such as methadone, decrease dose by 20 to 50 percent a day to 30 mg/day, then decrease 5 mg/day every 3 to 5 days to 10 mg/day, then decrease by 2.5 mg/day every 3 to 5 days; for Morphine CR, decrease dose by 20 to 50 percent a day to 45 mg/day, then decrease by 15 mg/day every 2 to 5 days; for Oxycodone CR, decrease by 20 to 50 percent a day to 30 mg/day, then decrease by 10 mg/day every 2 to 5 days; for fentanyl, first change to another opioid, such as morphine or methadone.[129] Note that when the letters CR follow a drug they stand for "controlled release," which means the drug is long acting and therefore does not need to be taken as frequently as the regular version of the drug.

Contact your doctor if you experience any withdrawal symptoms so your tapering regimen can be adjusted. These symptoms include cramping, anxiety, sweating, diarrhea, dilated pupils, goose bumps, increased blood pressure, insomnia, tearing of the eyes, muscle twitches, runny nose, increased heart rate, and increased breathing.

Another way to avoid withdrawal is to make sure that a new drug is not going to interfere with your current drugs. Other medications that can stimulate and/or block opioid receptors include nalbuphine (Nubain), buprenorphine (Buprenex, Subutex), naloxone (Narcan), buprenorphine/naloxone (Suboxone), pentazocine

(Talwin), pentazocine/naloxone (Talwin NX), naltrexone (Vivitrol), and nalmefene (Revex).[130] These medications should generally be avoided when taking opioid medications chronically. Knowing what your meds are for and the reality of what they can do will prevent an adverse event from occurring. Butorphanol (Stadol) blocks the effects of Wilmer's opioids and causes him to have an adverse event.

VIOLATION OF RULE #9: Be Aware of Drug Interactions

It is always a smart idea to talk to your pharmacist or doctor about how your medications work and whether they will interact with any medications you are currently taking. You can also look up drug interactions on your own at http://www.drugs.com. Take responsibility for your own safety, because the perfect system does not exist, and you need to be aware that your reactions are real.

VIOLATION OF RULE #14: Don't Stop Taking a Medication Without Talking to Your Doctor

Many medications can cause serious harm if stopped abruptly. In Wilmer's case, withdrawal occurs. Other problems can occur with other drugs, so it is wise to talk to your doctor before you stop taking them. Even if you believe you are having side effects from the medication, cannot afford the medication, or believe the medication is not working, do not discontinue your drugs without first talking to your doctor to determine why you were placed on the medication and to discuss the risks associated with stopping the drugs. This is especially the case with certain medications, such as opioids (such as fentanyl, Percocet, or morphine), benzodiazepines (such as diazepam [Valium], clonazepam [Klonopin], or alprazolam [Xanax]), and SSRIs (such as Zoloft, Prozac, or citalopram [Celexa]).

Conclusion

So there you are…you've just been given a guide to the top thirty dangerous intersections where your medications can collide. Now it is up to you to heed the warning signs. We know there are medications that are causing problems and aren't being reported or discussed with patients. This book alerts you to these interactions and gives you the knowledge you need to take precautions when using drugs.

Based on my training and years of experience, I am elated to share this knowledge that will help you become a better-informed patient and consumer of medications. Remember, slow down, know what to look out for, and proceed with caution. Don't let yourself become another statistic. We live in a society that often rushes quickly to add more medications when we don't feel well. Pay attention to your symptoms and remember to ask yourself: *Are Your Meds Making You Sick?*

Reader's Guide to Medications

One medication may be prescribed to patients with a variety of conditions, or a medication may produce a variety of side effects. That is why certain drugs are discussed in more than one chapter. To locate the drug that matches your health problem, look for the name of the medication in the left-most column of the alphabetical list in the special index. Then follow it across the columns to pinpoint the medical condition or symptom that concerns you most.

Medication	Body Area	Medical Condition/ Symptom	Chapter
Acetaminophen	Liver	Nausea, weakness	3, Medication-Induced Liver Dysfunction
Alcohol	Pancreas	Pain in abdomen	3, Medication-Induced Pancreatitis
Alendronate	Stomach, intestine	Abdominal pain, dizzy	5, Medication-Induced Gastrointestinal Ulceration
Amiodarone	Lung	Short of breath, coughing	2, Medication-Induced Lung Disease
Amoxicillin/ clavulinic acid	Intestine	Diarrhea	6, Medication-Induced Diarrhea
Aspirin	Stomach	Abdominal pain, weakness	5, Medication-Induced Upper-GI Bleeding
Calcium	Entire body	Lightheaded, dizzy	3, Medication-Induced Hypercalcemia
Carbamazepine	Brain	Seizure	4, Medication-Induced Seizure
Carisoprodol	Brain	Falling randomly	4, Medication-Induced Falls

(cont'd.)

Medication	Body Area	Medical Condition/ Symptom	Chapter
Digoxin	Entire body	Nausea, loss of appetite	4, Medication-Induced Digoxin Toxicity
Esitalopram	Entire body	Confused, shaking hands	4, Medication-Induced Serotonin Syndrome
Furosemide	Ears	Trouble hearing	4, Medication-Induced Hearing Loss
Etodolac	Kidney	Pain when urinating	3, Medication-Induced Liver Dysfunction
Fosinopril	Lung	Coughing	2, Medication-Induced Cough
Gemfibrozil	Legs	Pain in legs	6, Medication-Induced Rhabdomyolysis
Glyburide	Entire body	Confused, anxious	3, Medication-Induced Hypoglycemia
Hydrocodone	Lung	Difficulty breathing	2, Medication-Induced Respiratory Insufficiency
Insulin	Entire body	Sweaty, shaky	6, Medication-Induced Hypoglycemia
Levofloxacin	Heart	Irregular heart beat	2, Medicatio-Induced Arrhythmia
Lorazepam	Brain	Falling randomly	4, Medication-Induced Falls
Metformin	Entire body	Exhausted	6, Medication-Induced Lactic Acidosis
Metoclopramide	Left arm	Shaking left arm	6, Medication-Induced Movement Disorder
Mineral oil	Lung	Short of breath	2, Medication-Induced Pneumonia
Morphine	Lung	Difficulty breathing	2, Medication-Induced Respiratory Insufficiency
Nicotine (cigarettes)	Lung	Short of breath, coughing	2, Medication-Induced Lung Disease

(cont'd.)

Medication	Body Area	Medical Condition/ Symptom	Chapter
Oxycodone	Intestine	Constipation	5, Medication-Induced Intestinal Blockage
Phenytoin	Brain	Confused, upset stomach	4, Medication-Induced Change In Mental Status
Prednisone	Brain	Losing touch with reality	4, Medication-Induced Change In Mental Status
Ramipril	Entire body	Aches in legs	6, Medication-Induced Hyperkalemia
Simvastin	Legs	Pain in legs	6, Medication-Induced Rhabdomyolysis
Spironolactone	Entire body	Aches in legs	6, Medication-Induced Hyperkalemia
Sulfamethax/Tri-methoprim	Skin	Rash	6, Medication-Induced Stevens-Johnson Syndrome
Warfarin	Entire body	Bruising	5, Medication-Induced Subcutaneous Bleeding
Zolpidem	Brain	Falling randomly	4, Medication-Induced Falls

Notes

Introduction

1. Jason Lazarou, Bruce H. Pomeranz, and Paul N. Corey, "Incidence of Adverse Drug Reactions in Hospitalized Patients: A Meta-analysis of Prospective Studies," *Journal of the American Medical Association* 279 (1998): 1200–1205.
2. Ibid.
3. Jerry H. Gurwitz et al, "Incidence and Preventability of Adverse Drug Events among Older Persons in the Ambulatory Setting," *Journal of the American Medical Association* 289 (2003): 1107–1116; "Drug Reactions Kill Estimated 100,000 per Year," *CNN*, http://www.cnn.com/HEALTH/9804/14/drug.reaction (accessed 16 April 2008).
4. "Table 10. Number of Deaths from 113 Selected Causes by Age: United States, 2005," http://www.disastercenter.com/cdc/Age%20of%20Deaths%20113%20Causes%202005.html (accessed 25 May 2011).
5. Gurwitz et al, "Incidence and Preventability of Adverse Drug Events among Older Persons in the Ambulatory Setting."
6. Carla K. Johnson, "Fatal Medication Errors at Home Rise Rapidly," *Evansville Courier & Press* (29 July 2008).
7. T. J. Moore, M. R. Cohen, and C. D. Furberg, "Serious Adverse Drug Events Reported to the Food and Drug Administration, 1998–2005," *Archives of Internal Medicine* 167 (2007): 1752–1759.
8. "Medwatch—What Is a Serious Adverse Event?" *U.S. Food and Drug Administration*, http://www.fda.gov/safety/medwatch/howtoreport/ucm053087.htm (accessed 2 June 2011).
9. Lazarou, Pomeranz, and Corey, "Incidence of Adverse Drug Reactions in Hospitalized Patients," 1200–1205.
10. Kate King, "2008 Could Set Records for Tornado Deaths," *CNN*, http://www.cnn.com/2008/TECH/science/05/28/tornado.year/index.html (accessed 28 May 2008).

CHAPTER 1: The 16 Rules of Safe Medication Use

1. Kathleen Doheny, "Reports of Adverse Drug Effects Up: Increase Is

'Cause for Alarm,' Researchers Say," *WebMD Health News*, http:
//www.webmd.com/news/20070910/reports-of-adverse-drug
-effects-up (accessed 1 August 2008).

2. "FDA Accepts Adverse Drug Reaction Reports from Consumers," *Alliance for Human Research Protection*, http://www.ahrp.org/infomail
/0603/22.php (accessed 14 August 2008).

3. "FDA 101: How to Use the Consumer Complaint System and Med-
Watch," *U.S. Food and Drug Administration*, http://www.fda.gov/con
sumer/updates/reporting 061008.html (accessed 14 August 2008).

CHAPTER 2: Are Your Meds Causing Problems in the Lungs or Heart?

1. "Wikipedia, the Free Encyclopedia," *Wikipedia*, http://en.wikipedia
.org/wiki/Main_Page (accessed 8 August 2007); "Drug Name,"
Lexi-Drugs Online with AHFS, accessed via permission from http:
//www.lib.purdue.edu (accessed October–November 2007).

2. "State-Specific Prevalence of Current Cigarette Smoking among
Adults and Secondhand Smoke Rules and Policies in Homes and
Workplaces — United States, 2005," *Centers for Disease Control and
Prevention*, http://www.cdc.gov/mmwr/preview/mmwrhtml/mm
5542a2.htm (accessed 23 August 2007).

3. "Drugs, Herbs, and Supplements," *MedlinePlus*, http://www.nlm.nih
.gov/medlineplus/druginformation.html (accessed 8 August 2007);
"Prescription Drug Information, Side Effects, Interactions," *Drugs*,
http://www.drugs.com (accessed 8 August 2007); "Drug Name,"
Lexi-Drugs Online with AHFS; *Micromedex Healthcare Series* [Internet
database] (Greenwood Village, CO: Thomson Healthcare), updated
periodically.

4. "Wikipedia, the Free Encyclopedia," *Wikipedia*; "Drug Name," *Lexi-
Drugs Online with AHFS*.

5. G. L. Baum et al, eds., *Textbook of Pulmonary Diseases*, 6th ed. (Phila-
delphia: Lippincott-Raven, 1998), 837.

6. E. D. Chan, "Amiodarone Pulmonary Toxicity." In *UpToDate*, H. Holl-
ingsworth, ed. (Waltham, MA: UpToDate, 2008).

7. "Wikipedia, the Free Encyclopedia," *Wikipedia*.

8. Metin Ozkan, Raed A. Dweik, and Muzaffar Ahmad, "Drug-Induced
Lung Disease," *Cleveland Clinic Journal of Medicine* 68, no. 9 (2001):
782–95.

9. Ali Nawaz Khan, Klaus L. Irion, and Chitra P. Nagarajaiah, "Imaging in Drug-Induced Lung Disease," *eMedicine*, http://www.emedicine .com/radio/topic401.htm (accessed 15 August 2008).

10. "Top 200 Generic Drugs by Units in 2006," *Drug Topics*, http://www .drugtopics.com/drugtopics/data/articlestandard/drugtopics/092 007/407652/article.pdf (accessed 29 May 2006).

11. Baum et al, *Textbook of Pulmonary Diseases*, 837.

12. "Adverse Drug Reaction Electronic System," *Drug Safety Portal*, http: //www.adverse-drug-reaction.net/index.aspx (accessed February 2008–June 2008).

13. Matthew A. Silva et al, "Drug-Induced Pulmonary Toxicities," *U.S. Pharmacist* 32, no. 7 (2007): 48–54, http://uspharmacist.com/index .asp?show=article&page=8_2068.htm (accessed 15 August 2008).

14. *Micromedex Healthcare Series* [Internet database].

15. Silva et al, "Drug-Induced Pulmonary Toxicities."

16. "What Is a Serious Adverse Event?" *FDA*, http://www.fda.gov/mcd watch/report/DESK/advevnt.htm (accessed 2 June 2008); Lyle A. Siddoway, "Amiodarone: Guidelines for Use and Monitoring," *American Family Physician*, http://aafp.org/afp/20031201/2189.html (accessed 15 August 2008).

17. Richard Fogoros, "Amiodarone Lung Toxicity," *About.com: Heart Health Center*, http://heartdisease.about.com/od/drugsforheartdis ease/a/amiodarone_lung.html (accessed 4 August 2008).

18. Robin R. Hemphill, "Hypercalcemia," *eMedicine*, http://www.emedi cinc.com/emerg/topic260.htm (accessed 14 August 2008).

19. Uzkan, Ewelk, and Ahmad, "Lung Toxicity and Lung Disease."

20. *Micromedex Healthcare Series* [Internet database].

21. James E. Tisdale and Douglas A. Miller, *Drug-Induced Diseases—Prevention, Detection, and Management*, (Bethesda, MD: American Society of Health-System Pharmacists, 2005), p. 21.

22. "Drug Name," *Lexi-Drugs Online with AHFS*.

23. Ibid; "Drugs, Herbs, and Supplements," *MedlinePlus*, http://www.nlm .nih.gov/medlineplus/druginformation.html (accessed 25 August 2008).

24. Eyal Meltzer et al, "Lipoid Pneumonia: A Preventable Complication," *Israel Medical Association Journal* 8, no. 1 (2006): 33–35.

25. "Chemical Pneumonitis—Overview," *University of Maryland Medical Center*, http://www.umm.edu/ency/article/000143.htm (accessed 8 August 2008).

26. Meltzer et al, "Lipoid Pneumonia: A Preventable Complication."
27. Ibid.
28. Ibid.
29. Meltzer et al, "Lipoid Pneumonia: A Preventable Complication."
30. "Mineral Oil," *American Cancer Society,* http://www.cancer.org/doc root/CDG/content/CDG_mineral_oil.asp (accessed 4 August 2008).
31. Ibid.
32. Todd P. Selma, Judith L. Beizer, and Martin D. Higbee, *Lexi-Comp's Geriatric Dosage Handbook* (Hudson, OH: Lexi-Comp, Inc., 2003).
33. "Wikipedia, the Free Encyclopedia," *Wikipedia;* "Drug Name," *Lexi-Drugs Online with AHFS.*
34. Ibid.
35. Ibid.
36. C. M. White, "Drug-Induced Respiratory Depression," *U.S. Pharmacist,* http://www.uspharmacist.com/oldformat.asp?url=newlook /files/feat/acf2ece.cfm&pub_id=8&article_id=17.
37. White, "Drug-Induced Respiratory Depression."
38. "Adverse Drug Reaction Electronic System," *Drug Safety Portal.*
39. Sarah J. Johnson, "Opioid Safety in Patients with Renal or Hepatic Dysfunction," *Pain Treatment Topics,* http://pain-topics.org/pdf /Opioids-Renal-Hepatic-Dysfunction.pdf (accessed 4 August 2008); "Overdose," *Harm Reduction Coalition,* http://www.harmreduction .org/article.php?list=type&type=51 (accessed 4 August 2008).
40. "Overdose," *Harm Reduction Coalition.*
41. Selma, Beizer, and Higbee, *Lexi-Comp's Geriatric Dosage Handbook.*
42. "Safety Information for Using Morphine Sulphate," *Samaritan Pharmaceuticals,* http://www.samaritanpharma.com/morphine_sulphate /safety_information.asp (accessed 15 August 2008).
43. Selma, Beizer, and Higbee, *Lexi-Comp's Geriatric Dosage Handbook.*
44. "Safety Information for Using Morphine Sulphate," *Samaritan Pharmaceuticals.*
45. "Wikipedia, the Free Encyclopedia," *Wikipedia;* "Drug Name," *Lexi-Drugs Online with AHFS.*
46. Ibid.
47. Ibid.
48. N. M. Kaplan and B. D. Rose, "Major Side Effect of ACE Inhibitors." In *UpToDate,* A. M. Sheridan, ed. (Waltham, MA: UpToDate, 2008).

49. Silvestri, "Evaluation of Subacute and Chronic Cough in Adults."
50. "2004 Year-End U.S. Prescription and Sales Information and Commentary," *IMS*, http://www.imshealth.com/ims/portal/front/arti cleC/0,2777,6599_3665_69890098,00.html (accessed 23 January 2008).
51. "Top 200 Generic Drugs by Units in 2006," *Drug Topics*.
52. "U.S. and World Population Clocks," *U.S. Census Bureau*, http://www.census.gov/main/www/popclock.html (accessed 24 January 2008).
53. Silva et al, "Drug-Induced Pulmonary Toxicities."
54. Kaplan and Rose, "Major Side Effect of ACE Inhibitors."
55. "Incidence and Diagnosis of ACE-Induced Cough," *Medicines Management Network*, http://www.mmnetwork.nhs.uk/acaddetail/COU GHpercent20backgroundpercent20information.doc (accessed 22 January 2008).
56. "The Odds," *Funny2*, http://www.funny2.com/odds.htm (accessed 24 January 2008).
57. "Adverse Drug Reaction Electronic System," *Drug Safety Portal*.
58. Khan, Irion, and Nagarajaiah, "Imaging in Drug-Induced Lung Disease."
59. Silva et al, "Drug-Induced Pulmonary Toxicities."
60. Ozkan, Dweik, and Ahmad, "Drug-Induced Lung Disease."
61. "Wikipedia, the Free Encyclopedia," *Wikipedia*; "Drug Name," *Lexi-Drugs Online with AHFS*.
62. Ibid.
63. Ibid.
64. Jatin Dave and Revat Lakhia, "Torsades de Pointes," *eMedicine*, http://www.emedicine.com/med/topic2286.htm (accessed 26 February 2008); "Levofloxacin," *Facts and Comparison 4.0*, http://www2 .lib.purdue.edu (accessed 26 February 2008).
65. Dave and Lakhia, "Torsades de Pointes."
66. Ibid.; "The Heart Valves," *Texas Heart Institute*, http://www.texas heartinstitute.org/HIC/Anatomy/valves.cfm (accessed 26 February 2008).
67. Ibid.
68. Dave and Lakhia, "Torsades de Pointes."
69. Ibid.
70. Richard Frothingham, "Rates of Torsades de Pointes Associated with

Ciprofloxacin, Ofloxacin, Levofloxacin, Gatifloxacin, and Moxifloxacin," *Pharmacotherapy* 21, no. 12 (2001): 1468–72.

71. "Adverse Drug Reaction Electronic System," *Drug Safety Portal.*

72. "Levofloxacin," *Facts and Comparison 4.0*; "Drugs with Risk of Torsades de Pointes," *Arizona Center for Education and Research on Therapeutics*, http://www.torsades.org/medical-pros/drug-lists/list-01.cfm (accessed 7 August 2008).

73. Tisdale and Miller, *Drug-Induced Diseases—Prevention, Detection, and Management.*

74. Ibid.

CHAPTER 3: Are Your Meds Causing Kidney, Calcium, Liver, Pancreas, or Diabetic Complications?

1. "Drugs, Herbs, and Supplements," *MedlinePlus*, http://www.nlm.nih.gov/medlineplus/druginformation.html (accessed 8 August 2007); "Prescription Drug Information, Side Effects, Interactions," *Drugs.com*, http://www.drugs.com (accessed 8 August 2007); "Wikipedia, the Free Encyclopedia," *Wikipedia*, http://en.wikipedia.org/wiki/Main_Page (accessed 8 August 2007).

2. "Drug Name," *Lexi-Drugs Online with AHFS*, accessed via permission from http://www.lib.purdue.edu (accessed October–November 2007); *Micromedex Healthcare Series* [Internet database] (Greenwood Village, CO: Thomson Healthcare), updated periodically.

3. *Micromedex Healthcare Series* [Internet database].

4. "Drug Name," *Lexi-Drugs Online with AHFS*; *Micromedex Healthcare Series* [Internet database].

5. Ibid.

6. H. R. Howell, M. L. Brundige, and L. Langworthy, "Drug-Induced Acute Renal Failure," *U.S. Pharmacist* 32 (2007): 45–50; "Acute Renal Failure (ARF) Overview," *HealthCommunities.com*, http://www.nephrologychannel.com/arf (accessed 23 August 2007).

7. Ibid.

8. Ibid.

9. Loren Laine, "GI Effects of NSAIDs: Focus on Clinical Events," *Medscape Today*, http://www.medscape.com/viewarticle/561822_2 (accessed 13 August 2008).

10. Marie H. Pietruszka, "Drug-Induced Kidney Disease," *Journal of the*

Pharmacy Society of Wisconsin, http://www.pswi.org/meetings/ce /070807T.pdf (accessed 15 August 2008).

11. Guo Xiaoqing and Chike Nzerue, "How to Prevent, Recognize, and Treat Drug-Induced Nephrotoxicity," *Cleveland Clinic Journal of Medicine* 60, no. 4 (2002): 289–312.

12. "Adverse Drug Reaction Electronic System," *Drug Safety Portal,* http: //www.adverse-drug-reaction.net/index.aspx (accessed February 2008–June 2008).

13. Howell, Brundige, and Langworthy, "Drug-Induced Acute Renal Failure."

14. Tatyana Gurvich and Janet A. Cunningham, "Appropriate Use of Psychotropic Drugs in Nursing Homes," *American Family Physician,* http://www.aafp.org/afp/20000301/1437.html (accessed 11 August 2008).

15. Howell, Brundige, and Langworthy, "Drug-Induced Acute Renal Failure"; B. D. Rose and T. W. Post, "NSAIDs: Acute Renal Failure and Nephrotic Syndrome." In US Pharmacist.com (2007; 32(3):45–50), http://www.uspharmacist.com/content/d/featured%20articles /c/10379.

16. "How to Protect Your Kidneys," *The Kidney Trust,* https://www.kid neytrust.org/pykidneys.php (accessed 4 August 2008).

17. James E. Tisdale and Douglas A. Miller, *Drug-Induced Diseases — Prevention, Detection, and Management"* (Bethesda, MD: American Society of Health-System Pharmacists, 2005), 60.

18. Howell, Brundige, and Langworthy, "Drug-Induced Acute Renal Failure"; Rose and Post, "NSAIDs: Acute Renal Failure and Nephrotic Syndrome."

19. Howell, Brundige, and Langworthy, "Drug-Induced Acute Renal Failure"; Rose and Post, "NSAIDs: Acute Renal Failure and Nephrotic Syndrome."

20. "Drug Name," *Lexi-Drugs Online with AHFS; Micromedex Healthcare Series* [Internet database].

21. Ibid.

22. *Micromedex Healthcare Series* [Internet database]; "State-Specific Prevalence of Current Cigarette Smoking among Adults and Secondhand Smoke Rules and Policies in Homes and Workplaces — United States, 2005," *Centers for Disease Control and Prevention,* http://www

.cdc.gov/mmwr/preview/mmwrhtml/mm5542a2.htm (accessed 23 August 2007).

23. Robin R. Hemphill, "Hypercalcemia," *eMedicine*, http://www.emedi cine.com/emerg/topic260.htm (accessed 14 August 2008).

24. "Adverse Drug Reaction Electronic System," http://www.adverse -drug-reaction.net/index.aspx (accessed February 2008–June 2008).

25. Robin R. Hemphill, "Hypercalcemia," *eMedicine*, http://www.emedi cine.com/emerg/topic260.htm (accessed 14 August 2008).

26. Chris Woolston, "Heartburn: Symptoms and Treatment," *aHealthyMe!* http://www.ahealthyme.com/topic/heartburn (ac- cessed 4 August 2008).

27. *Micromedex Healthcare Series* [Internet database].

28. Ibid.

29. Ibid.

30. Germaine L. Defendi and Jeffrey R. Tucker, "Toxicity, Acetamino- phen," *eMedicine*, http://www.emedicine.com/ped/topic7.htm (ac- cessed 7 August 2008).

31. "Adverse Drug Reaction Electronic System," *Drug Safety Portal*; Maren Mayhew, "Acetaminophen Toxicity," *Journal for Nurse Practi- tioners* 3, no. 3 (2007): 186–88; A. Rahman Zamani, "Fact Sheets for Families: Acetaminophen Safety," *California Childcare Health Pro- gram*, http://www.ucsfchildcarehealth.org/pdfs/factsheets/acetamin en011804.pdf (accessed 8 August 2008); Ray Sahelian, "Acetamino- phen," *Dr. Ray Sahelian, M.D.*, http://www.raysahelian.com/aceta minophen.html (accessed 8 August 2008).

32. Defendi and Tucker, "Toxicity, Acetaminophen."

33. Susan E. Farrell, "Toxicity, Acetaminophen," *eMedicine*, http://www .emedicine.com/emerg/topic819.htm (accessed 15 August 2008).

34. Defendi and Tucker, "Toxicity, Acetaminophen."

35. "Drugs, Herbs, and Supplements, and Herbal Information," *Medline- Plus*; "Prescription Drug Information, Side Effects, Interactions," *Drugs.com*; "Wikipedia, the Free Encyclopedia," *Wikipedia*.

36. T. Gill and H. Polkinghorne, "Assessment and Treatment of Alco- hol Problems in the General Practice Setting," *NSW Department of Health*, http://www.health.nsw.gov.au/public-health/dpb/supple ments/supp3.pdf (accessed 23 August 2007).

37. "Alcohol Use," *Centers for Disease Control and Prevention*, http://www .cdc.gov/nchs/fastats/alcohol.htm (accessed 30 May 2007).

38. "Drug Name," *Lexi-Drugs Online with AHFS; Micromedex Healthcare Series* [Internet database].

39. Ibid.

40. "Drugs, Herbs, and Supplements, and Herbal Information," *Medline-Plus*; P. B. Kale-Pradhan and J. L. Conroy, "Pancreatitis." In *Drug-Induced Diseases: Prevention, Detection, and Management*, J. E. Tisdale and D. A. Miller, eds. (Bethesda, MD: ASHP, 2005), 537–47.

41. R. R. Berardi and P. A. Montgomery, "Pancreatitis." In *Pharmacotherapy: A Pathophysiologic Approach*, 6th ed., J. T. DiPiro et al, eds. (New York: McGraw-Hill, 2005), 729.

42. A. A. Fisher and M. L. Basset, "Acute Pancreatitis Associated with Angiotensin II Receptor Antagonists," *Annals of Pharmacotherapy* 36, no. 12 (2002): 1883–86.

43. P. G. Lankisch, M. Dröge, and F. Gottesleben, "Drug Induced Acute Pancreatitis: Incidence and Severity," *Gut* 37, no. 4 (1995): 565–67.

44. J. Granger and D. Remick, "Acute Pancreatitis: Models, Markers, and Mediators," *Shock* 24 (December 2005): 45–51.

45. M. C. Dufour and M. D. Adamson, "The Epidemiology of Alcohol-Induced Pancreatitis," *Pancreas* 27, no. 4 (November 2003): 286–90.

46. Tisdale and Miller, *Drug-Induced Diseases—Prevention, Detection, and Management*.

47. Robert S. Dinsmoor, "Lactic Acidosis," *Diabetes Self-Management*, http://www.diabetesselfmanagement.com/articles/Diabetes_Definitions/Lactic_Acidosis (accessed 6 August 2008); Rosalyn Carson-DeWitt, "Pancreatitis," *Healthline*, http://www.healthline.com/gale content/pancreatitis-1 (accessed 6 August 2008).

48. "Drug Name," *Lexi-Drugs Online with AHFS; Micromedex Healthcare Series* [Internet database].

49. Ibid.

50. Ibid.

51. Ibid.; R. I. Shorr et al, "Individual Sulfonylureas and Serious Hypoglycemia in Older People," *Journal of the American Geriatrics Society* 44, no. 7 (1996): 751–55.

52. "Adverse Drug Reaction Electronic System," *Drug Safety Portal*.

53. "Drug Name," *Lexi-Drugs Online with AHFS; Micromedex Healthcare Series* [Internet database]; Shorr et al, "Individual Sulfonylureas and Serious Hypoglycemia in Older People."

54. "All about Diabetes," *American Diabetes Association*, http://www.dia betes.org/about-diabetes.jsp (accessed 11 February 2008).

CHAPTER 4: Are Your Meds Playing Tricks with Your Mind?

1. "U.S. and World Population Clocks," *U.S. Census Bureau*, http://www .census.gov/main/www/popclock.html (accessed 1 November 2001).
2. "Top 200 Generic Drugs by Units in 2006," *Drug Topics*, http://www .drugtopics.com/drugtopics/data/articlestandard/drugtopics/092 007/407652/article.pdf (accessed 29 May 2006).
3. "Prescription Drug Information, Side Effects, Interactions," *Drugs .com*, http://www.drugs.com (accessed 8 August 2007).
4. Charlene A. Miller and Daniel M. Joyce, "Toxicity, Phenytoin," *eMedicine*, http://www.emedicine.com/emerg/topic421.htm (accessed 15 May 2007).
5. Thomas H. Glick, Tom P. Workman, and Slava V. Gaufberg, "Preventing Phenytoin Intoxication: Safer Use of a Familiar Anticonvulsant," *Journal of Family Practice*, http://www.jfponline.com/Pages.asp?AID =1656 (accessed 4 August 2008).
6. "Adverse Drug Reaction Electronic System," *Drug Safety Portal*, http: //www.adverse-drug-reaction.net/index.aspx (accessed February 2008–June 2008).
7. Miller and Joyce, "Toxicity, Phenytoin."
8. *Micromedex Healthcare Series* [Internet database] (Greenwood Village, CO: Thomson Healthcare), updated periodically.
9. "Drug Name," *Lexi-Drugs Online with AHFS*, accessed via permission from http://www.lib.purdue.edu (accessed October–November 2007); *Micromedex Healthcare Series* [Internet database].
10. Richard Hall, "Psychiatric Adverse Drug Reactions: Steroid Psychosis," *Dr. Richard C. W. Hall Publications*, http://www.drrichardhall .com/steroid.htm (accessed 1 August 2007).
11. "Drugs, Herbs, and Supplements," *MedlinePlus*, http://www.nlm.nih .gov/medlineplus/druginformation.html (accessed 8 August 2007); "Prescription Drug Information, Side Effects, Interactions," *Drugs .com*; "Wikipedia, the Free Encyclopedia," *Wikipedia*, http://en.wiki pedia.org/wiki/Main_Page (accessed 8 August 2007); "Drug Name," *Lexi-Drugs Online with AHFS*.
12. Kate King, "2008 Could Set Records for Tornado Deaths," *CNN*,

http://www.cnn.com/2008/TECH/science/05/28/tornado.year /index.html (accessed 28 May 2008).

13. Hall, "Psychiatric Adverse Drug Reactions: Steroid Psychosis."

14. *Micromedex Healthcare Series* [Internet database].

15. Hall, "Psychiatric Adverse Drug Reactions: Steroid Psychosis."

16. King, "2008 Could Set Records for Tornado Deaths."

17. Hall, "Psychiatric Adverse Drug Reactions: Steroid Psychosis."

18. Paul Perry and Brian C. Lund, "Steroid-Induced Mental Disturbances," *Virtual Hospital: Clinical Psychopharmacology Seminar*, http://www.tu .edu/user_files/10/27.html (accessed 4 August 2008).

19. Hall, "Psychiatric Adverse Drug Reactions: Steroid Psychosis."

20. Perry and Lund, "Steroid-Induced Mental Disturbances."

21. James E. Tisdale and Douglas A. Miller, *Drug-Induced Diseases — Prevention, Detection, and Management* (Bethesda, MD: American Society of Health-System Pharmacists, 2005).

22. Hall, "Psychiatric Adverse Drug Reactions: Steroid Psychosis."

23. "Drugs, Herbs, and Supplements," *MedlinePlus*; "Prescription Drug Information, Side Effects, Interactions," *Drugs.com*; "Wikipedia, the Free Encyclopedia," *Wikipedia*; "Drug Name," *Lexi-Drugs Online with AHFS*.

24. *Micromedex Healthcare Series* [Internet database].

25. "Drug-Induced Falls in the Elderly," *UIC College of Pharmacy Drug Information Center*, https://www.uic.edu/pharmacy/services/di/falls .htm (accessed 15 August 2008).

26. "Falls Among Older Adults: An Overview," *Centers for Disease Control and Prevention*, http://www.cdc.gov/ncipc/factsheets/adultfalls.htm (accessed 19 August 2007).

27. C. A. Wiens, "The Role of the Pharmacist in Falls Prevention in the Elderly," *Journal of Informed Pharmacotherapy* 6 (2001): 314–24.

28. "Adverse Drug Reaction Electronic System," *Drug Safety Portal*.

29. Joseph Woelfel, "Medication and Risk Factors That Lead to Falls," *Caring.com*, http://www.caring.com/articles/medication-and-risk -factors-that-lead-to-falls (accessed 5 August 2008); Natalie Brooks, "Medication and Falls in the Elderly," *Ontario Long Term Care Association*, http://www.oltca.com/Library/LTC/0308medication_falls .pdf (accessed 5 August 2008).

30. Woelfel, "Medication and Risk Factors That Lead to Falls."

31. Brooks, "Medication and Falls in the Elderly."

32. "Drug Name," *Lexi-Drugs Online with AHFS; Micromedex Healthcare Series* [Internet database].
33. John Hickey, "Risk of NSAIDS and GI Bleeding," *Just the Berries for Family Physicians,* http://www.theberries.ca/BOTW_archives/ns aids.html (accessed 29 October 2007).
34. "Drug Name," *Lexi-Drugs Online with AHFS; Micromedex Healthcare Series* [Internet database].
35. J. D. Lindh et al, "Incidence and Predictors of Severe Bleeding during Warfarin Treatment," *Journal of Thrombosis and Thrombolysis* 25, no. 2 (2008): 151–59, http://www.springerlink.com/content/877019w4t 535434k (accessed 31 October 2007).
36. "Drug Name," *Lexi-Drugs Online with AHFS; Micromedex Healthcare Series* [Internet database].
37. "Bipolar Disorder Alliance," *Depression and Bipolar Support Alliance,* http://www.dbsalliance.org (accessed 11 January 2008).
38. K. J. Kent, "Serotonin Syndrome." In *UpToDate,* J. Grayzel, ed. (Waltham, MA: UpToDate, 2008); "Neuroleptic Malignant Syndrome and Serotonin Syndrome: What Parents Must Know," *IMN,* http://www.imakenews.com/cabf/e_article000286683.cfm (accessed 29 January 2008); S. Nolan, "Serotonin Syndrome: Recognition and Management," *U.S. Pharmacist,* http://www.uspharmacist .com/oldformat.asp?url=newlook/files/feat/acg2fa6.htm (accessed 16 January 2008).
39. Kent, "Serotonin Syndrome."
40. Ibid.
41. Ibid.
42. Nolan, "Serotonin Syndrome: Recognition and Management."
43. B. D. Rose, "Manifestations of Hyponatremia and Hypernatremia." In *UpToDate,* T. W. Post, ed. (Waltham, MA: UpToDate, 2008).
44. "Adverse Drug Reaction Electronic System," *Drug Safety Portal.*
45. Kent, "Serotonin Syndrome."
46. Bettina C. Prator, "Serotonin Syndrome," *Journal of Neuroscience Nursing* 38, no. 2 (2006): 102–105, http://www.medscape.com/view article/547426_print135 (accessed 5 August 2008).
47. Nolan, "Serotonin Syndrome: Recognition and Management."
48. "Drug Name," *Lexi-Drugs Online with AHFS; Micromedex Healthcare Series* [Internet database].
49. "Drugs, Herbs, and Supplements," *MedlinePlus.*

50. "Drug Name," *Lexi-Drugs Online with AHFS; Micromedex Healthcare Series* [Internet database].

51. Ibid.

52. "Top 200 Generic Drugs by Units in 2006," *Drug Topics.*

53. Rose, "Manifestations of Hyponatremia and Hypernatremia"; G. M. Kuz and A. Manssourian, "Carbamazepine-Induced Hyponatremia: Assessment of Risk Factors," *Annals of Pharmacotherapy* 39, no. 11 (2005): 1943–46.

54. "Seizure Disorder," *Diablo Valley College,* http://www.dvc.edu/dss /faculty_staff_handbook/seizure_disorder.htm (accessed 21 January 2008).

55. C. M. Nzerue et al., "Predictors of Outcome in Hospitalized Patients with Severe Hyponatremia," *Journal of the National Medical Association* 95, no. 5 (2003): 335–43.

56. "Hyponatremia: Symptoms," *MayoClinic.com,* http://www.mayoclin ic.com/health/hyponatremia/DS00974/DSECTION=2 (accessed 21 January 2008).

57. Nzerue et al., "Predictors of Outcome in Hospitalized Patients with Severe Hyponatremia."

58. "Adverse Drug Reaction Electronic System," *Drug Safety Portal.*

59. "Hyponatremia: Symptoms," *MayoClinic.com.*

60. Tisdale and Miller, *Drug-Induced Diseases—Prevention, Detection, and Management.*

61. Mary Ann E. Zagaria, "Causes of Seizures in the Elderly," *U.S. Pharmacist* 33, no. 1 (2008): 27–31, http://www.uspharmacist.com/index .asp?show=article&page=8_2204.htm (accessed 15 August 2008).

62. "Drug Name," *Lexi-Drugs Online with AHFS; Micromedex Healthcare Series* [Internet database].

63. Ibid.

64. Ibid.

65. "2004 Year-End U.S. Prescription and Sales Information and Commentary," *IMS,* http://www.imshealth.com/ims/portal/front/arti cleC/0,2777,6599_3665_69890098,00.html (accessed 23 January 2008).

66. J. H. Wallace, "Digoxin Toxicity: A Review," *U.S. Pharmacist,* http: //www.uspharmacist.com/idex.asp?show=article&page=8_1694 .htm (accessed 24 January 2008); "Digitalis Toxicity and Fab Fragment," *Hamad Medical Corporation,* http://www.hmc.org.qa/qmj

/qmj_nov_2006/NOV2006/CONTINUOUS_M_E/Continous
ed.htm (accessed 28 January 2008).

67. Ibid.; N. Ismail, "Digitalis (Cardiac Glycoside) Intoxication." In
UpToDate, J. Grayzel, ed. (Waltham, MA: UpToDate, 2008); Lisa
Booze, "Digoxin Intoxication and the Use of Digoxin-Specific Fab
Antibody Fragments," http://64.233.169.104/search?q=cache:Iz1wI
80LSwUJ:http://www.mdpoison.com (accessed 28 January 2008).

68. Ibid.

69. Ibid.

70. Wallace, "Digoxin Toxicity: A Review."

71. K. M. Williamson et al, "Digoxin Toxicity: An Evaluation in Current
Clinical Practice," *Archives of Internal Medicine* 158, no. 22 (1998):
2444–49.

72. "Adverse Drug Reaction Electronic System," *Drug Safety Portal.*

73. "Digoxin, Lanoxin," *MedicineNet.com*, http://www.medicinenet.com
/digoxin/article.htm (accessed 5 August 2008).

74. Wallace, "Digoxin Toxicity: A Review."

75. "Drug Name," *Lexi-Drugs Online with AHFS*; *Micromedex Healthcare
Series* [Internet database].

76. "Top 200 Generic Drugs by Units in 2006," *Drug Topics.*

77. "Drug Name," *Lexi-Drugs Online with AHFS*; *Micromedex Healthcare
Series* [Internet database].

78. "Top 200 Generic Drugs by Units in 2006," *Drug Topics.*

79. "Drug Name," *Lexi-Drugs Online with AHFS*; *Micromedex Healthcare
Series* [Internet database].

80. W. S. Pray, "Ototoxic Medications," *U.S. Pharmacist* 19 (2005): 24–
29; *Micromedex Healthcare Series* [Internet database].

81. Pamela A. Mudd et al, "Inner Ear, Ototoxicity," *eMedicine*, http:
//www.emedicine.com/Ent/topic699.htm (accessed 25 June 2008).

82. "Adverse Drug Reaction Electronic System," *Drug Safety Portal.*

83. "Drugs, Herbs, and Supplements, and Herbal Information," *Medline-
Plus.*

84. Pray, "Ototoxic Medications."

85. Ibid.; Mudd et al, "Inner Ear, Ototoxicity."

CHAPTER 5: Are Your Meds Causing Bleeding Problems?

1. "Drug Name," *Lexi-Drugs Online with AHFS*, accessed via permission from http://www.lib.purdue.edu (accessed October–November

2007); *Micromedex Healthcare Series* [Internet database] (Green-wood Village, CO: Thomson Healthcare), updated periodically.

2. "Top 200 Generic Drugs by Units in 2006," *Drug Topics*, http://www.drugtopics.com/drugtopics/data/articlestandard/drugtopics/092 007/407652/article.pdf (accessed 29 May 2006).

3. "Drug Name," *Lexi-Drugs Online with AHFS; Micromedex Healthcare Series* [Internet database].

4. Ibid.

5. "Bleeding in the Digestive Tract," *National Digestive Diseases Information Clearinghouse*, http://digestive.niddk.nih.gov/ddiseases/pubs/bleeding (accessed 26 October 2007).

6. John Hickey, "Risk of NSAIDS and GI Bleeding," *Just the Berries for Family Physicians*, http://www.theberries.ca/BOTW_archives/ns aids.html (accessed 29 October 2007).

7. J. D. Lindh et al, "Incidence and Predictors of Severe Bleeding During Warfarin Treatment," *Journal of Thrombosis and Thrombolysis* 25, no. 2 (2008): 151–159, http://www.springerlink.com/content/877019w4t 535434k (accessed 31 October 2007).

8. J. Hollowell et al, "The Incidence of Bleeding Complications Associated with Warfarin Treatment in General Practice in the United Kingdom," *British Journal of General Practice* 53, no. 489 (2003): 312–14.

9. "Flash Facts about Lightning," *National Geographic News*, http://new s.nationalgeographic.com/news/2004/06/0623_040623_lightning fuatr html (accessed 1 November 2007).

10. "Adverse Drug Reaction Electronic System," *Drug Safety Portal*, http://www.adverse-drug-reaction.net/index.aspx (accessed February 2008–June 2008).

11. K. A. Valentine and R. D. Hull, "Outpatient Management of Oral Anticoagulation." In *UpToDate*, S. A. Landaw, ed. (Waltham, MA: UpTo-Date, 2008); "Patient Information: Warfarin (Coumadin)." *UpToDate*, http://patients.uptodate.com (accessed 22 October 2007).

12. "Drugs to Avoid while Taking Warfarin," *ACP Internist*, http://www.acponline.org/clinical_information/journals_publications/acp_in ternist/june06/drug_chart.pdf (accessed 6 August 2008).

13. "UW Health-Online Health Fact. INR and Stroke Prevention," *American Heart Association*, http://www.americanheart.org/down loadable/heart/1180475572009INR_StrokePrevention_patient _handout_UWMadison.pdf (accessed 6 August 2008).

14. "Drug Name," *Lexi-Drugs Online with AHFS; Micromedex Healthcare Series* [Internet database].

15. Ibid.

16. Ibid.

17. B. D. Rose, "Manifestations of Hyponatremia and Hypernatremia." In *UpToDate*, T. W. Post, ed. (Waltham, MA: UpToDate, 2008).

18. L. Laine, "Gastrointestinal Bleeding with Low-Dose Aspirin. What's the Risk? Gastrointestinal Bleeding in Randomized Controlled Trials of Low-Dose Aspirin for Cardiovascular Prevention," *American Journal of Gastroenterology* 95, no. 9 (2000): 2218–24, http://www.med scape.com/viewarticle/545101_3 (accessed 25 October 2007).

19. S. Nolan, "Serotonin Syndrome: Recognition and Management," *U.S. Pharmacist*, http://www.uspharmacist.com/oldformat.asp?url=new look/files/feat/acg2fa6.htm (accessed 16 January 2008).

20. James E. Tisdale and Douglas A. Miller, *Drug-Induced Diseases—Prevention, Detection, and Management*. (Bethesda, MD: American Society of Health-System Pharmacists, 2005), 67.

21. Ibid.

22. "Adverse Drug Reaction Electronic System," *Drug Safety Portal*.

23. J. A. Delaney et al, "Drug Drug Interactions Between Antithrombotic Medications and the Risk of Gastrointestinal Bleeding," *Canadian Medical Association Journal* 177, no. 4 (2007): 347–51.

24. Tisdale and Miller, *Drug-Induced Diseases—Prevention, Detection, and Management*.

25. "Gastrointestinal Bleeding with Low-Dose Aspirin," *American Journal of Gastroenterology*.

26. "Drug Name," *Lexi-Drugs Online with AHFS; Micromedex Healthcare Series* [Internet database].

27. Ibid.

28. "Hypothyroidism," *MedlinePlus*, http://www.nlm.nih.gov/medline plus/thyroiddisease.gov (accessed 11 January 2008).

29. "Drug Name," *Lexi-Drugs Online with AHFS; Micromedex Healthcare Series* [Internet database].

30. Fosamax (alendronate) package insert (Whitehouse Station, NJ: Merck, 2008).

31. "NSAIDs and Fosamax Are a Bad Brew," *Archives of Internal Medicine* 160, no. 5 (2000): 705–708; "NIH Consensus Statement 111, Osteo-

porosis, Prevention, Diagnosis, and Therapy," http://findarticles.com (accessed 29 October 2007).

32. Ibid.

33. Ibid.

34. Ibid.

35. "NSAID Gastrointestinal Adverse Effects," *FamilyPracticeNotebook. com*, http://fpnotebook.com/PHA44.htm (accessed 23 October 2007).

36. "U.S. and World Population Clocks," *U.S. Census Bureau*, http://www.census.gov/main/www/popclock.html (accessed 1 November 2001).

37. "NSAIDs and Fosamax Are a Bad Brew," *Archives of Internal Medicine*; "NIH Consensus Statement 111, Osteoporosis, Prevention, Diagnosis, and Therapy."

38. "Understanding GI Bleeding," *American College of Gastroenterology*, http://www.gi.org/patients/gibleeding/index.asp (accessed 29 October 2007).

39. Ibid.

40. "Adverse Drug Reaction Electronic System," *Drug Safety Portal*.

41. *Micromedex Healthcare Series* [Internet database].

CHAPTER 6: Are Your Meds Causing Strange and Unusual Symptoms?

1. "Drug 1...," *Peri-Drugs Online with AHFS*, accessed via permission from http://www.lib.purdue.edu (accessed October–November 2007); *Micromedex Healthcare Series* [Internet database] (Greenwood Village, CO: Thomson Healthcare), updated periodically.

2. Ibid.

3. "Constipation," *National Digestive Diseases Information Clearinghouse* http://digestive.niddk.nih.gov/ddiseases/pubs/constipation (accessed 13 January 2008).

4. Ibid.

5. "Drug Intelligence Brief," http://www.cesar.umd.edu/cesar/drugs /oxycodone.pdf (accessed 18 January 2008).

6. "Top 200 Generic Drugs by Units in 2006," *Drug Topics*, http://www .drugtopics.com/drugtopics/data/articlestandard/drugtopics/092 007/407652/article.pdf (accessed 29 May 2006).

7. "Constipation," *National Digestive Diseases Information Clearinghouse.*

8. Clyde R. Goodheart and Stewart B. Leavitt, "Managing Opioid-Induced Constipation in Ambulatory-Care Patients," *Pain Treatment Topics,* http://pain-topics.org/pdf/Managing_Opioid-Induced_Con stipation.pdf (accessed 6 August 2008).

9. "Constipation," *National Digestive Diseases Information Clearinghouse.*

10. S. J. Panchal, P. Müller-Schwefe, and J. I. Wurzelmann, "Opioid-Induced Bowel Dysfunction: Prevalence, Pathophysiology, and Burden," *International Journal of Clinical Practice* 61, no. 7 (2007): 1181–1187.

11. James E. Tisdale and Douglas A. Miller, *Drug-Induced Diseases—Prevention, Detection, and Management* (Bethesda, MD: American Society of Health-System Pharmacists, 2005), 122.

12. "Adverse Drug Reaction Electronic System," *Drug Safety Portal,* http://www.adverse-drug-reaction.net/index.aspx (accessed February 2008–June 2008).

13. Goodheart and Leavitt, "Managing Opioid Induced Constipation in Ambulatory-Care Patients."

14. Ibid.

15. "Drug Name," *Lexi-Drugs Online with AHFS; Micromedex Healthcare Series* [Internet database].

16. "Hypothyroidism," *MedlinePlus,* http://www.nlm.nih.gov/medline plus/thyroiddisease.gov (accessed 11 January 2008).

17. "Drug Name," *Lexi-Drugs Online with AHFS; Micromedex Healthcare Series* [Internet database].

18. T. Gill and H. Polkinghorne, "Assessment and Treatment of Alcohol Problems in the General Practice Setting," *NSW Department of Health,* http://www.health.nsw.gov.au/public-health/dpb/supple ments/supp3.pdf (accessed 23 August 2007).

19. "Alcohol Use," *Centers for Disease Control and Prevention,* http://www .cdc.gov/nchs/fastats/alcohol.htm (accessed 30 May 2007).

20. "Metformin-Associated Lactic Acidosis," *Medscape Today,* http://www.medscape.com/viewarticle/417792_3 (accessed 8 February 2008); Metformin Hydrochloride, package insert, *Covidien,* http://pharmaceuticals.mallinckrodt.com; Kyle J. Gunnerson and Sat Sharma, "Lactic Acidosis," *eMedicine,* http://www.emedicine.com /MED/topic1253.htm (accessed 8 February 2008).

21. Ibid.

22. Ibid.

23. Ibid.

24. Robert S. Dinsmoor, "Lactic Acidosis," *Diabetes Self-Management,* http://www.diabetesselfmanagement.com/articles/Diabetes_Definitions/Lactic_Acidosis (accessed 6 August 2008).

25. "Adverse Drug Reaction Electronic System," *Drug Safety Portal.*

26. "Metformin," *DiabetesNet.com,* http://www.diabetesnet.com/diabetes_treatments/metformin.php (accessed 7 February 2008); "Hypoglycemia," *National Diabetes Information Clearinghouse,* http://diabetes.niddk.nih.gov/dm/pubs/hypoglycemia/index.htm#remember (accessed 7 February 2008).

27. P. Pillans, "Metformin and Fatal Lactic Acidosis," *Medsafe,* http://www.medsafe.govt.nz/Profs/PUarticles/5.htm (accessed 6 August 2008).

28. "Drug Name," *Lexi-Drugs Online with AHFS; Micromedex Healthcare Series* [Internet database].

29. Ibid.

30. Ibid.

31. Ibid.

32. "Hypoglycemia," *National Diabetes Information Clearinghouse.*

33. Ibid.; "All about Diabetes," *American Diabetes Association,* http://www.diabetes.org/about-diabetes.jsp (accessed 11 February 2008).

34. Ibid.

35. Metin Ozkan, Raed A. Dweik, and Muzaffar Ahmad, "Drug-Induced Lung Disease," *Cleveland Clinic Journal of Medicine* 68, no. 9 (2001): 782–95.

36. "Drug Intelligence Brief," http://www.cesar.umd.edu/cesar/drugs/oxycodone.asp (accessed 18 January 2008).

37. "Travelers' Diarrhea," *Centers for Disease Control and Prevention,* http://www.cdc.gov/ncidod/dbmd/diseaseinfo/travelersdiarrhea_g.htm (accessed 26 February 2008).

38. Steven J. Parrillo and Catherine V. Parrillo, "Stevens-Johnson Syndrome," *eMedicine,* http://www.emedicine.com/emerg/topic555.htm (accessed 26 February 2008).

39. "Drug Name," *Lexi-Drugs Online with AHFS; Micromedex Healthcare Series* [Internet database].

40. Ibid.

41. Ibid.

42. Parrillo and Parrillo, "Stevens-Johnson Syndrome"; "Erythema

Multi-forme," *Uniformed Services University of the Health Sciences,* http://rad.usuhs.mil/derm/lecture_notes/Images/EM_palm.jpg (accessed 26 February 2008).

43. Parrillo and Parrillo, "Stevens-Johnson Syndrome."

44. Ibid.; "Bactrim," *Facts and Comparison 4.0,* http://www2.lib.purdue .edu (accessed 26 February 2008).

45. Parrillo and Parrillo, "Stevens-Johnson Syndrome."

46. "Adverse Drug Reaction Electronic System," *Drug Safety Portal.*

47. D. S. Budnitz et al, "National Surveillance of Emergency Department Visits for Outpatient Adverse Drug Events," *Journal of the American Medical Association* 296, no. 15 (2006): 1858–66; Marian Wald Myers and Hershel Jick, "Hospitalization for Serious Blood and Skin Disorders Following Use of Co-Trimoxazole," *British Journal of Clinical Pharmacology* 43, no. 4 (1997): 446–48.

48. J. C. Roujeau et al, "Medication Use and the Risk of Stevens-Johnson Syndrome or Toxic Epidermal Necrolysis," *New England Journal of Medicine* 333, no. 24 (1995): 1600–1607; Heather Brannon, "Help, I Have a Rash," *About.com: Dermatology,* http://dermatology.about .com/cs/miscellaneous/a/rash.htm (accessed 26 February 2008).

49. Roujeau et al, "Medication Use and the Risk of Stevens-Johnson Syndrome or Toxic Epidermal Necrolysis."

50. Brannon, "Help, I Have a Rash."

51. "Drug Name," *Lexi-Drugs Online with AHFS; Micromedex Healthcare Series* [Internet database].

52. Ibid.

53. Ibid.

54. K. A. Antons et al, "Clinical Perspectives of Statin-Induced Rhabdomyolysis," *American Journal of Medicine* 119, no. 5 (2006): 400–409; "Rhabdomyolysis," *MedlinePlus,* http://www.nlm.nih.gov/medline plus/ency/article/000473.htm (accessed 20 February 2008).

55. "Rhabdomyolysis," *MedlinePlus*; "Simvastatin," *Facts and Comparisons 4.0,* http://www2.lib.purdue.edu (accessed 20 February 2008).

56. Antons et al, "Clinical Perspectives of Statin-Induced Rhabdomyolysis"; "Rhabdomyolysis," *MedlinePlus*; "Simvastatin," *Facts and Comparisons 4.0.*

57. Ibid.

58. "Rhabdomyolysis," *MedlinePlus.*

59. Antons et al, "Clinical Perspectives of Statin-Induced Rhabdomyolysis"; "Simvastatin," *Facts and Comparisons 4.0.*
60. Tisdale and Miller, *Drug-Induced Diseases—Prevention, Detection, and Management.*
61. Brannon, "Help, I Have a Rash."
62. "Adverse Drug Reaction Electronic System," *Drug Safety Portal.*
63. Antons et al, "Clinical Perspectives of Statin-Induced Rhabdomyolysis"; "Rhabdomyolysis," *MedlinePlus*; "Simvastatin," *Facts and Comparisons 4.0.*
64. Tisdale and Miller, *Drug-Induced Diseases—Prevention, Detection, and Management.*
65. Ibid.
66. "Top 200 Brand Drugs by Units in 2007," *Drug Topics,* http://www.nxtbook.com/nxtbooks/advanstar/dt021808/index.php (accessed 14 August 2008).
67. "Drug Name," *Lexi-Drugs Online with AHFS; Micromedex Healthcare Series* [Internet database].
68. "Top 200 Generic Drugs by Units in 2006," *Drug Topics.*
69. "Drug Name," *Lexi-Drugs Online with AHFS; Micromedex Healthcare Series* [Internet database].
70. Ibid.
71. M. A. Zagaria, "Risk in Clinical Trials vs. Clinical Practice," *U.S. Pharmacist* 11 (2004): 29–34; David N. Juurlink et al, "Rates of Hyperkalemia after Publication of the Randomized Aldactone Evaluation Study," *New England Journal of Medicine* 351, no. 6 (2004): 543–51.
72. Ibid.
73. Ibid.
74. Zagaria, "Risk in Clinical Trials vs. Clinical Practice."
75. "Adverse Drug Reaction Electronic System," *Drug Safety Portal.*
76. "Top 200 Generic Drugs by Units in 2006," *Drug Topics.*
77. "Hyperkalemia Induced by Aldosterone Antagonists," *Medscape,* http://www.medscape.com/viewarticle/521319_6 (accessed 17 June 2008).
78. "Drug Name," Lexi-Drugs Online with AHFS; Micromedex Healthcare Series [Internet database].
79. Ibid.
80. Ibid.

81. "Top 200 Generic Drugs by Units in 2006," *Drug Topics.*

82. "An Update on the Changing Epidemiology and Treatment of *Clostridium difficile*–Associated Diarrhea," *U.S. Pharmacist*, http://www.uspharmacist.com/index.asp?show=article&page=8_1766.htm; C. P. Kelly, C. Pothoulakis, and J. T. LaMont, "*Clostridium difficile* Colitis," *New England Journal of Medicine* 330, no. 4 (1994): 257–62.

83. Ibid.

84. "Rhabdomyolysis," *MedlinePlus.*

85. Tisdale and Miller, *Drug-Induced Diseases—Prevention, Detection, and Management.*

86. Michael S. Schroeder, "*Clostridium difficile*–Associated Diarrhea," *American Family Physician*, http://www.aafp.org/afp/20050301/921.html; M. L. Job and N. F. Jacobs, Jr., "Drug-Induced *Clostridium difficile*-Associated Disease," *Drug Safety* 17, no. 1 (1997): 37–46.

87. Job and Jacobs, "Drug-Induced *Clostridium difficile*–Associated Disease."

88. Tisdale and Miller, *Drug-Induced Diseases—Prevention, Detection, and Management.*

89. "Adverse Drug Reaction Electronic System," *Drug Safety Portal.*

90. Kelly, Pothoulakis, and LaMont, "*Clostridium difficile* Colitis."

91. J. R. McDonald, "Prevention and Control of *Clostridium difficile* in Hospital and Institutional Settings." In *UpToDate*, E. L. Baron, ed. (Waltham, MA: UpToDate, 2008).

92. Tisdale and Miller, *Drug-Induced Diseases—Prevention, Detection, and Management.*

93. "Drug Name," *Lexi-Drugs Online with AHFS; Micromedex Healthcare Series* [Internet database].

94. Ibid.

95. Ibid.

96. Ibid.

97. Ibid.; L. Ganzini et al, "The Prevalence of Metoclopramide-Induced Tardive Dyskinesia and Acute Extrapyramidal Movement Disorders," *Archives of Internal Medicine* 153, no. 12 (1993): 1469–1475.

98. Ganzini et al, "The Prevalence of Metoclopramide-Induced Tardive Dyskinesia and Acute Extrapyramidal Movement Disorders," 1469–1475.

99. "Metoclopramide Hydrochloride," *Mosby's Drug Consult*, http://www

.mosbysdrugconsult.com/DrugConsult/Top_200/Drugs/e1798
.html (accessed 6 August 2008).

100. "Adverse Drug Reaction Electronic System," *Drug Safety Portal*.

101. Tatyana Gurvich and Janet A. Cunningham, "Appropriate Use of Psychotropic Drugs in Nursing Homes," *American Family Physician*, http://www.aafp.org/afp/20000301/1437.html (accessed 11 August 2008).

102. Tisdale and Miller, *Drug-Induced Diseases—Prevention, Detection, and Management*.

103. Ibid.

104. "Metoclopramide Hydrochloride," *Mosby's Drug Consult*.

105. Tisdale and Miller, *Drug-Induced Diseases—Prevention, Detection, and Management*.

106. Gurvich and Cunningham, "Appropriate Use of Psychotropic Drugs in Nursing Homes."

107. Tisdale and Miller, *Drug-Induced Diseases—Prevention, Detection, and Management*.

108. "Drug Name," *Lexi-Drugs Online with AHFS; Micromedex Healthcare Series* [Internet database].

109. Ibid.

110. Ibid.

111. Olivera J. Bogunovic and Shelly F. Greenfield, "Practical Geriatrics: Use of Benzodiazepines among Elderly Patients," *Psychiatric Services*, http://www.psychservices.psychiatryonline.org/cgi/content/full/55/3/233 (accessed 31 July 2008).

112. "The Beers List: Potentially Inappropriate Medications for the Elderly," *Duke Clinical Research Institute*, https://www.dcri.org/trial-par ticipation/the-beers-list (accessed 31 July 2008).

113. Robin Mantooth, "Toxicity, Benzodiazepine," *eMedicine*, http://www.emedicine.com/emerg/topic58.htm (accessed 30 July 2008).

114. "Adverse Drug Reaction Electronic System," *Drug Safety Portal*.

115. *5 Million Lives Campaign Getting Started Kit: Prevent Adverse Drug Events (Medication Reconciliation) How-to-Guide* (Cambridge, MA: Institute for Healthcare Improvement, 2008), http://www.ihi.org.

116. "Top 200 Generic Drugs by Units in 2006," *Drug Topics*.

117. G. Rogers et al. "Reconciling Medications at Admission: Safe Practice Recommendations and Implementation Strategies." *Joint Commission Journal on Quality and Patient Safety* 32 (2006): 37–50.

118. *5 Million Lives Campaign Getting Started Kit.*

119. Gurvich and Cunningham, "Appropriate Use of Psychotropic Drugs in Nursing Homes."

120. Todd P. Selma, Judith L. Beizer, and Martin D. Higbee, *Lexi-Comp's Geriatric Dosage Handbook* (Hudson, OH: Lexi-Comp, Inc., 2003).

121. "Drug Name," *Lexi-Drugs Online with AHFS; Micromedex Healthcare Series* [Internet database].

122. Ibid.

123. "Stadol NS, package insert," *National Migraine Association*, http://www.migraines.org/treatment/pdfs/Stadol03.pdf (accessed 31 July 2008).

124. "Adverse Drug Reaction Electronic System," *Drug Safety Portal.*

125. "Critical Review of Butorphanol," *World Health Organization*, 34th ECDD, http://www.who.int/medicines/areas/quality_safety/4.1Bu thorphanolCritReview.pdf (accessed 1 August 2008).

126. "Top 200 Generic Drugs by Units in 2006," *Drug Topics.*

127. "Top 200 Generic Drugs by Retail Sales in 2003," *Drug Topics*, http://drugtopics.modernmedicine.com/drug topics/article/article Detail.jsp?id=104567 (accessed 31 July 2008).

128. "Top 200 Generic Drugs by Units in 2007," *Drug Topics.*

129. Lee A. Kral, "Opioid Tapering: Safely Discontinuing Opioid Analgesics," *Pain Treatment Topics*, http://pain-topics.org/pdf/Safely_Taper ing_Opioids.pdf (accessed 8 August 2008).

130. *Micromedex Healthcare Series* [Internet database].

Glossary

A good first place to look up definitions of medical terms is the MedlinePlus website at http://www.nlm.nih.gov/medlineplus/mplusdictionary.html.

ACE inhibitors. *See* angiotensin converting enzyme (ACE) inhibitors.

angiotensin converting enzyme (ACE) inhibitors. Used to decrease blood pressure.

acute. Severe, sudden onset.

acute respiratory distress syndrome (ARDS). A life-threatening lung condition that prevents enough oxygen from getting into the blood.

ADR. *See* adverse drug reaction.

adrenal insufficiency. An endocrine disorder that occurs when the adrenal glands do not produce enough of certain hormones.

adverse drug reaction. An injury resulting from the use of a drug.

alanine transaminase (ALT). An enzyme found in the highest quantities in the liver. Injury to the liver results in the release of this enzyme into the blood.

albumin. A protein made by the liver.

alkaline phosphate (Alk Phos). An enzyme whose levels are tested to detect liver disease or bone disorders. When damaged, liver cells release an increased amount of alkaline phosphate into the blood.

Alk Phos. *See* alkaline phosphate.

ALT. *See* alanine transaminase.

anaerobic. Without oxygen.

analgesic. Used to control pain.

anemia. A condition in which blood does not carry enough oxygen to the rest of the body.

angiotensin receptor blockers (ARB). A class of medications to reduce blood pressure.

anion gap. An increase in the levels of this value often suggests the presence of too much acid, which can occur as a result of drug poisoning or kidney failure.

antiarrhythmics. A class of medications used to treat irregular heart rhythm.

259

antibiotic. A class of medications used to treat infection.

antimuscarinic. Blocking the muscarinic receptors.

antipyretic. A class of medications used to treat fever.

aplastic anemia. A blood disorder in which the body's bone marrow does not make enough new blood cells.

ARB. *See* angiotensin receptor blockers.

ARDS. *See* acute respiratory distress syndrome.

arrhythmia. A change in rhythm of the heart.

aspiration pneumonia. Caused by breathing foreign materials (food, liquid, vomit) into the lungs, which, in turn, causes a lung infection (pneumonia).

aspartate aminotransferase (AST). An enzyme found in high amounts in heart muscle and the liver.

AST. *See* aspartate aminotransferase.

ataxia. A failure of muscular coordination.

benzodiazepine. A class of medications used to treat anxiety.

bilirubin. A test used to measure liver function; high levels indicate a liver disorder.

black box label. A type of warning that appears on the package insert for medications that can have side effects or cause serious adverse effects. It is named for the black border that surrounds the text of the warning.

blood urea nitrogen (BUN). A test that, when elevated, may indicate that the kidneys are not working well.

bronchioles. Small tubes in the lung system.

bronchiolitis. A common illness of the respiratory tract caused by an infection that affects the tiny airways of the lungs.

bronchitis. An inflammation of the bronchial tubes.

BSA. The abbreviation for body surface area.

BUN. *See* blood urea nitrogen.

calcium channel blockers. A class of medications used to treat high blood pressure.

cardiogenic shock. A state in which a suddenly weakened heart is not able to pump enough blood to meet the body's needs. The condition is a medical emergency and is fatal if not treated quickly.

cardiovascular. Involving the heart and blood vessels.

central nervous system depression. A condition in which the central nervous system is depressed, which can result in a decreased rate of breathing, decreased heart rate, and loss of consciousness, possibly leading to death or coma.

chemical pneumonitis. An inflammation of the lungs or breathing difficulty due to inhaling chemical fumes or breathing in and choking on certain chemicals.

chemotherapy. A process of using a class of medications to treat cancer.

chest radiograph. An X ray of the chest.

cilia. Hairlike projections in the bronchus in the lungs that move debris up and out of the airways.

Clostridium difficile. Bacteria that cause diarrhea and a more serious intestinal condition that affects the colon.

cognition. The process of being aware, knowing, thinking, and judging.

contraindicated. Indicating the inadvisability of a medication.

controlled substance. Any medication that is regulated by state and federal laws that aim to control the danger of addiction, abuse, and physical and mental harm.

chronic obstructive pulmonary disease (COPD). A chronic lung disease.

corticosteroids. A group of steroids used to treat inflammation.

COX II inhibitors. A class of medications that are a form of nonsteroidal anti-inflammatory drugs that target COX-2, an enzyme responsible for inflammation and pain.

computerized axial tomography (CT scan). A test that provides very clear pictures of the interior of the body.

COPD. *See* chronic obstructive pulmonary disease.

CT scan. *See* computerized axial tomography.

diabetes type 1. Diabetes means blood glucose is too high. With type 1 diabetes, the pancreas does not make insulin.

diabetes type 2. Diabetes means blood glucose is too high. With type 2 diabetes, the pancreas makes insufficient levels of insulin.

digestive. The function of digesting food.

digoxin. A medication used to treat heart failure and irregular heartbeats.

digoxin toxicity. Toxicity caused by too much digoxin.

diuretic. A class of medications that help the body get rid of extra fluid.

diffusion capacity of lung for carbon monoxide (DLCO). Measures how well the lungs exchange gases.

DLCO. *See* diffusion capacity of lung for carbon monoxide.

drug dosages. The amount of medication administered to a patient. Don't be confused by drug dosages—they depend on the actual potency of the drug in question. Depending on potency, some medications are in grams, some in milligrams, and some in micrograms. One gram is equal to 1,000 milligrams. One milligram is equal to 1,000 micrograms.

dysfunction. A disturbance or impairment.

dyskinesia. Impairment of voluntary movement.

dyspepsia. Impairment of digestion.

edema. Swelling of body areas caused by excessive fluids.

electrolytes. Salts in the body fluids that are important to the function of the body, such as sodium, potassium, and calcium.

emphysema. A progressive disease of the lungs, usually caused by smoking.

fulminant. A condition that occurs suddenly and with great intensity.

gastrointestinal reflex disease (GERD). Occurs when a muscle at the end of the esophagus does not close properly, allowing the stomach contents to leak back into the esophagus.

gastroparesis. Paralysis of the stomach; it can occur in diabetes.

glomerular filtration rate (GFR). Used to measure kidney function.

gastrointestinal (GI) tract bleeding. Any bleeding that starts in the gastrointestinal tract, which extends from the mouth to the anus.

GERD. *See* gastrointestinal reflex disease.

GFR. *See* glomerular filtration rate.

glucocorticoids. A type of steroids used to treat inflammation.

glycated hemoglobin (HgA1C). A lab test and a form of hemoglobin used primarily to identify the average plasma glucose concentration over prolonged periods of time.

gout. A common form of arthritis that causes swollen and painful joints.

HDL. *See* high-density lipoprotein.

HgA1C. *See* glycated hemoglobin.

H2 blocker. A class of medications (also called H2 receptor blockers) that reduce the amount of acid the stomach produces by blocking histamine.

high-density lipoprotein (HDL). Also known as the "good" cholesterol.

heart failure. A condition in which the heart has lost the ability to pump enough blood to the body's tissues.

heart block. Refers to a delay in the normal flow of electrical impulse that causes the heart to beat.

hepatic. Having to do with the liver.

hypercalcemia. A condition that indicates high calcium.

hyperkalemia. A condition that indicates high potassium.

hypertension. A condition that indicates high blood pressure.

hypoglycemia. A condition that indicates low blood glucose.

hypotension. A condition that indicates low blood pressure.

hypothyroidism. A state in which the thyroid's hormone production is below normal.

infiltrate. To penetrate.

inflammation. A localized protective response elicited by injury.

international normalized ratio (INR). A lab test that measures blood clotting. INR is used to monitor warfarin levels.

insulin. Produced by the pancreas to let the body use glucose effectively.

interstitial pneumonitis. A form of lung disease characterized by progressive scarring of both lungs.

lab values. A term that describes the numerical value of laboratory test results that fall within a defined range (particularly important for evaluating kidney and liver function).

lactic acidosis. A condition of too much acid in the body due to the buildup of lactic acid.

LDL. *See* low-density lipoprotein.

low-density lipoprotein (LDL). Also known as the "bad" cholesterol.

leukopenia. A decreased white blood cell count resulting from many different situations, such as chemotherapy or radiation therapy.

lipids. A group of fats and fatlike substances.

lipoid pneumonia. A specific form of lung inflammation (pneumonia) that develops when lipids enter the lungs.

malabsorption syndrome. A condition that occurs when the small intestine cannot absorb nutrients from foods.

MAOI. *See* monoamine oxidase inhibitor.

monoamine oxidase inhibitor (MAOI). A group of antidepressant medications that inhibit the action of monoamine oxidase in the brain.

mcg/mL. Micrograms per milliliter of fluid—a concentration of substance per milliliter.

medication reconciliation. A formal process of identifying the most accurate list of medications a patient is taking.

megaloblastic anemia. A blood disorder in which anemia with elevated levels of red blood cells is present.

mEq/L. Milliequivalent per liter—a concentration of substance per liter.

metabolism. A process by which the liver changes the drug to be excreted by the body.

metabolite. A substance produced by the process of metabolism.

monitoring parameters. A set of labs results or vital signs to monitor the effectiveness of a medication.

myasthenia gravis. An autoimmune neuromuscular disease that leads to muscle weakness and fatigue.

myocardial infarction. A heart attack.

myopathy. Muscle disease.

narcotic. A natural or synthetic drug that acts like morphine.

narrow therapeutic index. If a drug has a narrow therapeutic index that means the blood level required to be effective is close to the level that causes significant side effects and/or toxicity.

neurological. Having to do with the nerves or the nervous system.

neutropenia. Low neutrophil count. Neutrophils are immature white blood cells.

noxious. Harmful to living things.

nonsteroidal anti-inflammatory drugs (NSAIDs). A group of medications that treat pain or inflammation.

NSAIDS. *See* nonsteroidal anti-inflammatory drugs.

opiate. A medication derived from opium.

opioid. A narcotic that has opiate-like actions (pain relieving) but is not derived from opium.

ototoxic. Damaging to the ear.

palliative. A treatment that seeks to treat symptoms.

pancreatitis. A disease in which the pancreas becomes inflamed.

pancytopenia. A shortage of all types of blood cells.

peripheral vascular disease. A disease of blood vessels outside the heart.

peristalsis. The rippling motion of muscles in the digestive tract.

photosensitivity. Sensitivity to light.

pneumonia. An inflammation of the lungs, usually caused by an infection.

pneumonitis. Inflammation of the lungs.

PPIs. *See* proton pump inhibitors.

proton pump inhibitors (PPIs). A group of medications that block the proton pump and are used in gastroesophageal reflux disease.

proactive. Acting in advance to deal with an expected difficulty.

proarrhythmic. Having a tendency to cause an irregular heart rate.

psychosis. Any severe mental disorder in which contact with reality is lost or highly distorted.

psychotropic. A group of medications that affect the mind, mood, or other mental processes.

pulmonary. Pertaining to the lungs.

pulmonary fibrosis. The formation or development of excess fibrous connective tissue in the lungs.

pulmonary function tests. Evaluate how much air the lungs can hold and can help diagnose lung disease.

QT interval. A measurement of the heart's electrical cycle. A prolonged QT interval increases the chance of ventricular tachyarrhythmia.

reference range. A set of values that are considered normal for an individual.

renal. Pertaining to the kidneys.

respiratory depression. Slowing of the breathing rate.

respiratory insufficiency. Insufficient breathing for proper bodily function.

rhabdomyolysis. The breakdown of skeletal muscle due to injury.

sedation. State of reduced excitement.

seizure. The physical findings or changes in behavior that occur after an episode of abnormal electrical activity in the brain.

serotonin syndrome. A condition that occurs when medications that cause high levels of the chemical serotonin accumulate in the body.

serum creatinine (SCr). A test that reveals important information about the kidneys. An elevated creatinine test indicates poor kidney function.

SCr. *See* serum creatinine.

selective serotonin reuptake inhibitors. A commonly prescribed type of antidepressant.

SSRI. Abbreviation for selective serotonin reuptake inhibitors.

serum Kl-6/MUC1. A lab test to determine whether a patient has interstitial pneumonitis.

somnolence. Drowsiness.

stevens-johnson syndrome. A condition in which the skin and mucous membranes react severely to a medication or infection.

supraventricular tachycardia. An abnormally fast heartbeat caused by rapid electrical impulses.

therapeutic range. The blood level of a drug that corresponds to an effective response.

thrombocytopenia. A condition that indicates a low number of platelets in the blood.

thyroid function tests. Determine the health of the thyroid gland.

torsades de pointes. A dangerous ventricular irregular heart rhythm that may cause passing out or sudden death.

toxic epidural necrolysis. A skin disorder due to an allergic reaction or infection.

toxicity. The level at which a medication can become harmful.

tremors. Unintentional trembling or shaking movements in one or more parts of the body.

triglycerides. A type of fat. Levels of triglycerides are checked in a lab to determine the amount of fat in the bloodstream and fat tissue.

ulceration. Development of an ulcer.

urine output. The amount of urine produced by the kidneys.

ventricular dysfunction. An abnormal pumping of the ventricles of the heart.

vertigo. Dizziness.

Important Web Resources

Beers Criteria for Potentially Inappropriate Medication Use in the Elderly
http://www.dcri.duke.edu/ccge/curtis/beers.html
Includes a list of medications that the elderly should generally avoid.

Drugs.com   http://www.drugs.com
Drug information for prescription, over-the-counter, and natural products.

Epocrates   http://www.epocrates.com
Drug information one can access concerning drug dosages and adverse events from medications.

FDA Adverse Event Reporting System
https://www.prosoftedc.com/aers.html
Look up adverse events that may result from the use of various medications.

FDA Medwatch Website
http://www.fda.gov/medwatch/report/consumer/consumer.htm
Report problems that you think may be associated with your medications.

Medline Plus
http://www.nlm.nih.gov/medlineplus/mplusdictionary.html
A medical dictionary.

Globalrph.com   http://www.globalrph.com
Drug information on mechanism of action and drug dose adjustments.

Medscape   www.medscape.com
Information on drug uses, dosages, and side effects.

FDA drug list   http://www.accessdata.fda.gov/scripts/cder/drugsatfda
Drugs listed by names, strength, and generic name.

WebMD   http://www.webmd.com/drugs
A database of drugs and warnings.

My Medicine Record

In the United States we have a big problem with medicines being prescribed from multiple sources by people unaware that the patient may already be taking another drug that will interact poorly with what they are prescribing. This problem can easily be prevented if each person keeps an accurate listing of all OTC and prescription drugs they are taking at a given moment and makes sure all of their doctors and pharmacists are given a copy. To help you do this, here is a template (see the next page) that you can use to track the following information for each drug you are taking: the drug's name, what it looks like, your dosage, how and when to take it, when you should start and stop taking it, why you are taking it, and who prescribed or suggested it.

MY MEDICINE RECORD

Name (Last, First, Middle Initial): _____   Birth Date (mm/dd/yyyy): _____

	What I'm Using (Rx—Brand and generic name; OTC—Name and active ingredients)	What It Looks Like (color, shape, size, markings, etc.)	How Much	How to Use/When to Use	Start/Stop Dates	Why I'm Using/Notes	Who Told Me to Use/How to Contact
1							
2							
3							

These are my medicines as of (Enter date as mm/dd/yyyy): _____

(Source: www.fda.gov/Drugs/ResourcesForYou/ucm079489.htm / [888] INFO-FDA / www.fda.gov/usemedicinesafely / FORM FDA 3664 [3/11])

A blank copy of this form may be downloaded from the entry for this book at www.hunterhouse.com.

Index

A

Accupril (quinapril), 45–46, 108
ACE (angiotensin-converting enzyme)
inhibitors: coughing, 44–50; drug
names, 45, 201; elderly patient tolerance, 48; fetus development warnings, 32–33, 46, 152; hyperkalemia,
200–204; overview of properties,
45–46; pancreatitis, 83; renal dysfunction, 64; sales statistics, 47–48
acetaminophen (Tylenol): adverse drug
reaction rating, 13; advertisements and
public information, 79; as alternative
pain medication, 62, 64, 69, 70, 155–
156; breathing problems, 40–41, 44;
drug interactions, 15, 73, 79, 143;
falling risks, 108; liver dysfunction, 74–
79; overdose statistics, 76; overview,
73, 131, 218; pancreatitis, 83. See also
hydrocodone/acetaminophen
N-acetylcysteine, 75
acetylsalicylic acid (aspirin), 83, 135, 143,
146–151, 175
ACTH (adrenocorticotropic hormone),
101
Actonel (risedronate), 155
acyclovir, 64
Adalat (nifedipine), 108, 182
adverse drug reactions (ADRs), overview: death statistics, 1, 4; definition,
2; emergency-room statistics, 1, 4;
prevention of, 8; reporting of, 2, 6–8,
23; safety determination rules, 13–22
Adverse Event Reporting System, 11
advertisements, 22–23, 79, 159, 197–198
Advil (ibuprofen), 46, 83, 135, 157, 159
age, and drug tolerance, 15–16
albuterol, 98–99
alcohol: consumption limitation recommendations, 84; consumption statis-

tics, 80; drug interaction warnings,
15, 73, 79, 144, 199; falling, 107; lactic
acidosis, 170, 172, 173; overview, 80,
168; pancreatitis, 81–84; risk awareness, 18, 84; seizures, 122
alcohol-containing medications, 107
Aldactone (spironolactone), 198–199,
201–204
Aldomet (methyldopa), 83
aldosterone antagonists, 201, 202
alendronate, 151–159
Aleve (naproxen), 67, 69, 70, 153–159
Alka Seltzer, 70–71
allopurinol, 64, 187
alprazolam (Xanax), 107, 211, 230
Altace (ramipril), 45–46, 118, 199–204
amantadine, 115
Ambien (zolpidem), 104–105
American Association of Poison Control
Centers, 76
amikacin, 135
aminoglycosides, 64, 135
aminopenicillins, 187
amiodarone, 25–31, 56, 96, 128, 143
amitriptyline (Elavil), 107, 115, 216
amlodipine, 59–60, 61
amoxicillin (Amoxil), 187, 208
amoxicillin/clavulanic acid (Augmentin),
187, 205–210
Amoxil (amoxicillin), 187, 208
amphetamines, 115
amphotericin B, 64
ampicillin, 208
Anafranil (clomipramine), 115, 216
analgesics. See acetaminophen; hydroco-
done/acetaminophen; nonsteroidal
anti-inflammatory drugs; pain medications
anemia, 150
angina medications, 124–125, 205

angiotensin-converting enzyme inhibitors. *See* ACE (angiotensin-converting enzyme) inhibitors
angiotensin receptor blockers (ARBs), 49–50, 64, 80–81, 202
anorexia, 126
antacids, 67–72
antiallergy medications, 107
antiandrogens, 199
antianxiety medications, 32, 104–107, 190–191, 199, 211, 218–224, 230
antiarrhythmics, 25–31, 56
antibiotics, 52–57, 83, 85, 115, 182–189, 205–210
anticoagulants, 156–157
anticonvulsants, 108, 121, 186
antidepressants: citalopram, 190–191, 230; duloxetine, 93, 94; escitalopram, 110–116; falling risks, 107; mirtazapine, 92; seizures, 122; serotonin syndrome, 115; trazodone, 60, 63, 115; withdrawal issues, 230
antiepileptics, 83, 187
antifungal agents, 197
antigout medications, 187
antihistamines, 107
antimuscarinic agents, 216
antineoplastics, 3, 135
antipsychotics, 107, 122, 211, 215
antiseizure medications: carbamazepine, 77–78, 117–118, 120–122, 186, 187, 216; falling risks, 108; phenytoin, 64, 78, 92–97, 108, 117, 187
antitestosterone steroids, 199
ARBs (angiotensin receptor blockers), 49–50, 64, 80–81, 202
arrhythmia, 50–57, 124, 182
Artane (trihexyphenidyl), 108, 216
arthritis medications, 59, 60–65, 130–131, 133, 134, 157
ASA (acetylsalicylic acid, aspirin), 83, 135, 143, 146–151, 175
aspirin, 83, 135, 143, 146–151, 175
asthma medications, 98–103, 187
Atacand (candesartan), 81, 202
Atarax (hydroxyzine), 107

atenolol (Tenormin), 108, 205
Ativan (lorazepam), 32, 104–107
atorvastatin (Lipitor), 147, 194, 197
Augmentin (amoxicillin/clavulanate potassium), 187, 205–210
Avalide (irbesartan), 49, 81, 202
Avelox (moxifloxacin), 55, 187
azathioprine, 83
Azilect (rasagiline), 108, 191
azithromycin, 143, 197, 208

B

Bactrim (sulfamethoxazole/trimethoprim), 143, 182–187
Benadryl, 107
benazepril, 38, 39–40, 201
Bentyl (dicyclomine), 108
benzodiazepine antagonists, 221
benzodiazepines: clonazepam, 218–224, 230; decreasing risk of falling, 107; diazepam, 199, 219–224, 230; falling risks, 224; hospitalization statistics, 220; lorazepam, 32, 104–107; withdrawal, 230
benztropine, 216
bepridil, 56
beverages, 144, 182. *See also* alcohol
bipolar disorder, 101, 109–116
bisacodyl, 165, 166
bisphosphonates, 155, 156
bleeding: common signs of, 143, 150, 157–158; drug–herb interactions causing, 18; gastrointestinal ulcerations, 151–159; hospitalization statistics, 141–142; overview, 136; subcutaneous (bruising), 136–145; upper-gastrointestinal, 145–151
blood clotting reduction medications. *See* aspirin; warfarin
blood pressure medications: amlodipine, 59–60, 61; atenolol, 108, 205; benazepril, 38, 39–40; enalapril/hydrochlorothiazide, 152, 201; falling risks, 108; fosinopril, 45–50, 108, 201; lisinopril, 32–34, 83, 108, 201; losartan, 49, 80–81, 82, 202; metoprolol, 26, 51;

potassium loss, promoting, 201–202; ramipril, 45–46, 118, 199–204. *See also* ACE inhibitors; ARBs; furosemide
blood sugar, low, 174–180
blood urea nitrogen (BUN), 14
Boniva (ibandronate), 155
breathing problems, 37–44
bromocriptine (Parlodel), 108, 115
bronchitis, chronic, 28
bruising, 136–145
bumetanide, 135
Buprenex (buprenorphine hydrochloride), 229
buprenorphine/naloxone, 229
buprenorphine, 229
bupropion (Wellbutrin), 115, 122
buspirone (Buspar), 107, 115
butorphanol, 226–230

C
caffeine, 182
Calan (verapamil), 108
calcium carbonate, 66–72
calcium channel blockers (CCBs), 59–60
calcium excess, 66–72
candesartan (Atacand), 81, 202
captopril (Capoten), 45, 48, 108
carbamazepine (Carbatrol, Tegretol, Tegretol XR): acetaminophen byproduct production, 77–78; movement disorders, 216; overview, 117–118; seizures, 120–122; Stevens-Johnson Syndrome, 186, 187
carboplatin, 135
Cardizem (diltiazem), 108
carisoprodol (Soma), 104–107
Catapres (clonidine), 108
CAT (computerized axial tomography) scans, 27
CBC (complete blood count), 118, 122
CCBs (calcium channel blockers), 59–60
CDAD (*Clostridium difficile*–associated diarrhea), 204–210
Ceftin (cefuroxime), 187
cefuroxime, 187
Celebrex (celecoxib), 130–131, 133, 134, 157

celecoxib, 130–131, 133, 134, 157
Celexa (citalopram), 115, 190–191, 230
Centers for Disease Control and Prevention (CDC), 42
cephalexin (Keflex), 187
cephalosporins, 187, 208
chemotherapy drugs, 3, 135
chest pain medications, 124–125, 205
chloroquine, 56, 135
chlorpromazine (Thorazine), 56, 108, 122, 216
cholesterol-control medications, 45, 67, 147, 190–198, 205
cholesterol panels, 195–196
cigarette smoking, 25, 27–28, 29, 99
cimetidine, 71, 168, 170
ciprofloxacin (Cipro), 55, 143, 187, 208
cisapride, 56
cisplatin, 3, 64, 135
citalopram (Celexa), 115, 190–191, 230
clarithromycin, 56, 143
clavulanic acid/amoxicillin, 205–210
clindamycin, 208
clinical trials, 7, 60, 154
clomipramine, 115, 216
clonazepam, 218–224, 230
clonidine (Catapres), 108
clorazepate (Tranxene), 107
Clostridium difficile–associated diarrhea (CDAD), 204–210
clotrimazole, 197
clozapine (Clozaril), 108, 122
Clozaril (clozapine), 108, 122
cocaine, 115
codeine, 108, 115, 164
Colace (docusate), 35, 36, 162, 163, 165
commercials, 22–23, 79, 159, 197–198
Compazine (prochlorperazine), 108, 211–215, 216
confusion, 110, 174
congenital anomaly, 2
constipation, 162, 163–165
COPD, 170
Cordarone (amiodarone), 25–31, 56, 96, 128, 143
corticosteroids, 83, 98–103, 149, 156, 187
cortisone, 101

coughing, 44–50
cough medicines, 107
Coumadin (warfarin), 13, 18, 36, 96, 136–145, 149, 182
Cozaar (losartan), 49, 80–81, 82, 202
cranberry juice, 144
creatinine, 61
creatinine kinase (CK), 191–192, 195
cyclobenzaprine (Flexeril), 108
cyclosporine, 64, 197
Cymbalta (duloxetine), 93, 94

D
Dalmane (flurazepam), 107, 108
death statistics, 1, 4, 42, 75, 114, 168, 221
dehydration, 61–62, 173, 203, 209, 210
delirium, 101, 221
Deltasone (prednisone), 99–103, 187
Demadex (torsemide), 108
Demerol (meperidine), 3–4, 5, 115, 122
Depakene/Depakote (valproic acid), 83, 96, 108, 120, 187
depression, 101, 109–110
desipramine (Norpramin), 107, 115
Desyrel (trazodone), 60, 63, 115
Detrol (tolterodine), 108
dextromethorphan, 115
diabetes: blood sugar levels, normal, 176–177; consequences of, 163, 165; medications for, 86, 147, 175, 176; patient education, 179, 180
diabetic medications: diabetic complications due to, 84–90; emergency-room visits, 13; falling, 108; herbal products as, 182; hypoglycemia, 174–180; lactic acidosis, 167–168, 169–173; seizures, 122
diarrhea, 204–210
Diaßeta (glyburide), 86–90, 108, 147
diazepam (Valium), 107, 199, 219–224, 230
diclofenac, 135, 157
dicyclomine (Bentyl), 108
digoxin (Digitek, Lanoxin, Lanoxicaps), 123–129, 137–138
Dilantin (phenytoin), 64, 78, 92–97, 108, 117, 187, 216

diltiazem (Cardizem), 108
Diovan (valsartan), 49, 81, 202
diphenhydramine, 216
discontinuation of medication, 20, 22, 26, 224–230
disopyramide, 56
Ditropan (oxybutynin), 108
diuretics: enalapril/hydrochlorothiazide, 152, 201; hearing risks, 135; hydrochlorothiazide, 51, 54, 82, 83, 202; hyponatremia, 121; potassium-sparing, 201; renal dysfunction, 64. *See also* furosemide
docusate, 35, 36, 162, 163, 165
dofetilide, 56
Donnatal (belladonna/phenobarbital), 108
doom, sense of, 40–41
dopamine agonists, 115
dopamine blockers, 161, 211, 213–214
dosage: adverse reactions caused by incorrect, 18–19; corticosteroid therapy and, 102; and elderly patients, 22, 36, 43–44, 216, 220–221, 224; manufacturer recommendations, 19; prescription compliance *vs.* self-dosing, 16, 71, 84–90, 158
doxepin (Sinequan), 107, 115, 216
droperidol, 56, 216
duloxetine (Cymbalta), 93, 94
Duragesic (fentanyl), 115, 164, 225, 227–230
Dyazide (triamterene and hydrochlorothiazide), 108

E
effectiveness, 16–17
Effexor (venlafaxine), 115
Elavil (amitriptyline), 107, 115, 216
elderly patients: ACE inhibitor reactions, 48; aspirin recommendations, 175; and constipation, 162; digoxin toxicity, 128; dosage guidelines, 22, 36, 43–44, 166, 216, 220–221, 224; falling, 106–107; inappropriate medication lists for, 220–221; medication tolerance awareness, 15–16, 57, 166; seizures, 122; ulceration, 149

emergency-room visits: acetaminophen toxicity, 78; digoxin toxicity, 128–129; drug safety and statistical awareness of, 13–14; insulin misuse, 180; statistics, 1, 4; sulfonamide-containing antibiotic reactions, 186; warfarin toxicity, 144
emphysema, 27–28, 171
Emsam (selegiline), 191
enalapril (Vasotec), 45–46, 83, 108, 152
enalapril/hydrochlorothiazide, 152, 201
erythromycin, 56, 83, 143, 197, 208
escitalopram, 110, 113–116
Eskalith (lithium), 64, 111–116, 115, 122
esomeprazole (Nexium), 71
estazolam, 107
estrogens, 83
ethacrynic acid, 135
ethosuximide (Zarontin), 96, 108
etodolac, 59, 60–65, 135
ezetimibe, 205
ezetimibe/simvastatin, 45, 67

F
falling, 103–109, 129, 144, 221, 224
famotidine, 168
fasting blood sugar (FBS), 176
fecal impaction, 160–166
Felbatol (felbamate), 108
fenofibrate (Tricor), 195, 197
fenoprofen, 135
fentanyl (Duragesic, Fentora), 115, 164, 225, 227–230
fibrates, 190–194
Flagyl (metronidazole), 83, 143, 207
Flexeril (cyclobenzaprine), 108
Floxin (ofloxacin), 55
flumazenil, 221
fluoxetine (Prozac), 115, 230
flurazepam (Dalmane), 107, 108
Food and Drug Administration (FDA), 1, 2, 7, 11. See also MedWatch
Fosamax (alendronate), 151–159
fosinopril (Monopril), 45–50, 108, 201
Furadantin (nitrofurantoin), 83
furosemide (Lasix): falling risks, 108; hearing loss, 132–135; herbal product interactions, 182; overview, 123–124,

131, 137; pancreatitis, 83; potassium-loss promotion, 201–202

G
gabapentin (Neurontin), 108
gastric stasis medication, 161
gastric ulcer medications, 168, 170
gastroesophageal reflux disease (GERD) medications, 168, 170
gastrointestinal antispasmodics, 107, 108
gastrointestinal bleeding, 145–151
gastrointestinal reflux medication, 161
gastrointestinal tract, defined, 148
gastrointestinal ulcerations, 151–159
gastroparesis, 36, 163
gatifloxacin, 55
gemfibrozil (Lopid), 190–194
gentamicin, 135
GFR (glomerular filtration rate), 42
ginko biloba, 18
ginseng, 18, 115, 182
Glucophage (metformin), 108, 167–168, 169–173
glyburide (Diaßeta, Glynase, PresTab, Micronase), 86–90, 108, 147
grapefruit juice, 144
guidelines for medications, 5–6

H
Halcion, 107
Haldol, 108
hallucinations, 98–103, 124
haloperidol, 56, 216
halos around lights, 123, 126
H2 blockers, 71
hearing loss, 130–135
heartburn, 152
heartburn medications, 70–71, 211, 213–214
heart function, 50–57, 123–129
heart medications: arrhythmia, 56; bleeding, 138–145, 149; and emergency-room statistics, 13; falling, 129; herbal-product interactions, 18, 182; lung disease, 25–31; overview of function, 138–139; toxicity caused by, 123–129
hepatotoxity. See liver dysfunction and damage

herbal products, 18, 114, 115, 165, 166, 182
hospitalists, 6
hospitalizations, 127, 149, 156, 202, 220.
    See also emergency-room visits
Humulin R (insulin), 175, 177–180
hydrochlorothiazide, 51, 54, 82, 83, 108,
    202
hydrochlorothiazide/enalapril, 152, 201
hydrocodone/acetaminophen (Lortab,
    Vicodin, Norco): falling risks, 108;
    liver-damage statistics, 76; overview,
    38, 73–74, 225–226; respiratory insuf-
    ficiency, 40–41, 44
HydroDiuril (hydrochlorothiazide), 108
hydromorphone, 164
hydroxyzine (Atarax), 107
hypercalcemia, 66–72
hyperkalemia, 198–204
hypoglycemia, 86, 88–89, 174–180
hypoglycemic medications, 108
hypokalemia, 54
hyponatremia, 118–122
hypothyroidism, 111

I

ibandronate (Boniva), 155
ibuprofen (Advil, Motrin), 46, 83, 135,
    137, 159
ibutilide, 56
identification, medical, 144
Imdur (isosorbide), 124–125
imipramine (Tofranil), 107, 115
immunosuppressant medications, 83
Inderal (propranolol), 108
INRs (international normalized ratios),
    136–137, 140–141, 142, 145
insulin, 13, 108, 122, 174–180
insulin glargine, 176, 178
insulin regular, 175, 177–180
interactions, drug: awareness, 17–18; bev-
    erages, 144; bleeding, 143, 156–157;
    decrease absorption, 36; digoxin
    toxicity, 125; herbal products, 18, 182;
    opioid receptor interference, 229–230,
    230; rhabdomyolysis/myopathy,
    192–193, 196–197; seizures, 122;
    serotonin syndrome, 114–116

international normalized ratios (INRs),
    136–137, 140–141, 142, 145
intestinal blockage, 160–166
irbesartan (Avalide), 49, 81, 202
Ismo (isosorbide), 124–125
isocarboxazid (Marplan), 43, 115, 191
isoniazid, 78, 122
Isoptin (verapamil), 108
isosorbide mononitrate, 124–125
itraconazole, 143

J

Jantoven (warfarin), 13, 18, 36, 96,
    136–145, 149, 182
Joint Commission, 5, 19, 222

K

K (vitamin), 141, 143
kanamycin, 135
Kayexalate (sodium polystyrene sulfo-
    nate), 201
Keflex (cephalexin), 187
ketoconazole, 143, 197
kidney (renal) function: chemotherapy
    drugs affecting, 3; digoxin toxicity and,
    123, 125, 126, 129; diuretics and hear-
    ing loss, 133–134; hyperkalemia and,
    202, 203; lab value awareness, 14–15,
    42, 43, 65, 89, 129, 173, 203; lactic
    acidosis, 171, 172; medication-induced
    kidney failure, 58–65; rhabdomyolysis
    effects on, 193
Klonopin (clonazepam), 218–224, 230
Kondremul, 33, 34–36

L

lab testing: cholesterol panels, 195–196;
    complete blood counts (CBCs), 118,
    122, 158; international normalized
    ratios (INRs), 136–137, 140–141, 142,
    145; kidney, 14–15, 42, 43, 65, 89,
    129, 173, 203; lab values and refer-
    ence ranges, 14–15; liver, 15, 75, 78,
    122, 195; lung function, 31; potassium
    levels, 204; schedule adherence, 16
lactic acidosis, 167–173
lamotrigine, 187

Lanoxicaps/Lanoxin (digoxin), 123–129, 137–138
lansoprazole, 151, 216
Lantus, 176, 178
Lasix. *See* furosemide
laxatives, 33, 34–36, 162, 165, 166
levodopa, 115, 216
levofloxacin (Levaquin), 52–57, 143, 187, 208
levothyroxine (Synthroid, Levothroid, Levoxyl, Unithroid), 111
Levsin (hyoscyamine), 108
Lexapro (escitalopram), 110, 113–116
Librax (chlordiazepoxide and clidinium), 108
lidocaine, 121, 122
linezolid, 115
lipid panels, 195–196
Lipitor (atorvastatin), 147, 194, 197
Liqui-Doss, 33, 34–36
lisinopril (Prinivil), 32–34, 83, 108, 201
lithium (Eskalith, Lithobid), 64, 111–116, 115, 122
liver dysfunction and damage: heartburn medications causing, 71; lab-value monitoring, 15, 75, 78, 122, 195; lactic acidosis, 173; pain killers causing, 13, 72–79; phases of, 76–77; toxicity statistics, 75–76
liver enzyme tests, 195–196
liver transplantation, 75, 76
Lodine (etodolac), 59, 60–65, 135
Lopid (gemfibrozil), 190–194
Lopressor (metoprolol), 26, 51
lorazepam (Ativan), 32, 104–107
Lortab. *See* hydrocodone/acetaminophen
losartan, 49, 80–81, 82, 202
Lotensin (benazepril), 38, 39–40, 201
lovastatin, 194
loxapine (Loxitane), 108
Loxitane (loxapine), 108
LSD, 115
lung disease, 24–36, 171. *See also* pneumonia

M
Maalox, 71
Macrobid (nitrofurantoin), 85

macrolides, 197, 208
mania, 101, 109–113
MAOIs (monoamine oxidase inhibitors), 45, 115, 191
Marplan (isocarboxazid), 43, 115, 191
Maxzide (triamterene and hydrochlorothiazide), 108
medical records, 2, 6, 17–18, 19–20, 114, 217–224
medication lists, 19–20, 21, 223
MedWatch: arrhythmia, 55; benzodiazepine, 221; *C. diff* colitis, 208; constipation, 164; consumer reporting at, 7–8, 23; falling, 106; gastrointestinal bleeding, 149, 157; hallucination, 101; hypercalcemia, 69; hyponatremia, 121; INR elevation, 142; lactic acidosis, 171; liver damage and transplantation, 76; lung disease, 30; movement disorder, 214; opiate withdrawal, 228; ototoxicity, 134; physician reports, 23; respiratory depression, 41; rhabdomyolysis, 194; serotonin syndrome, 114; Stevens-Johnson Syndrome, 186
Mellaril (thioridazine), 108
mental status changes, 91–97, 98–103, 217–220, 221
meperidine, 3–4, 5, 115, 122
mesoridazine, 56
metaxalone (Skelaxin), 108, 199
metformin (Glucophage), 108, 167–168, 169–173
methadone, 56, 164
methotrexate, 64
methyldopa, 83
metoclopramide (Reglan), 108, 161, 211, 213–214, 216
metolazone (Zaroxolyn), 108
metoprolol, 26, 51
metronidazole, 83, 143, 207
Micardis (telmisartan), 49, 81, 202
Micronase (glyburide), 86–90, 108, 147
Microzide (hydrochlorothiazide), 51, 54, 82, 83, 202
mineral oil, 33, 34–36
Mirapex (pramipexole), 108
mirtazapine, 92

moexipril, 45–46, 201, 202
monitoring parameters, 16–17, 65, 72, 145, 180, 196
monoamine oxidase inhibitors (MAOIs), 108, 115, 191
Monoket (isosorbide), 124–125
Monopril (fosinopril), 45–50, 108, 201
morphine, extended release (MS Contin), 3, 4, 37–38, 40–42, 164, 230
Motrin (ibuprofen), 46, 83, 135, 157
movement disorders, 210–216
moxifloxacin, 55, 187
MS Contin (morphine, extended release), 3, 4, 37–38, 40–42, 164, 230
mucosa, 184
muscle pain, 147, 170, 189–198
muscle relaxants, 104–107, 199
muscle weakness, 189–198
Mylanta, 71
myopathy, 189–198

N
nalbuphine, 229
nalmefene, 230
naloxone, 229
naloxone/buprenophine, 229
naloxone/pentazocine, 230
naltrexone, 230
NAPQI, 75
naproxen (Aleve, Naprosyn), 67, 69, 70, 135, 153–159
Narcan (naloxone), 229
Nardil (phenelzine), 43, 115, 191
narrow therapeutic indexes, 124
National Patient Safety Goals, 5, 222
nausea-relief medications, 161, 211–215
Navane (thiothixene), 108
NebuPent (pentamidine), 56, 83
nefazodone, 115
Nembutal (pentobarbital), 108
neomycin, 135
Neupro (rotigotine), 108
Neurontin (gabapentin), 108
Nexium (esomeprazole), 71
nicotine, 25, 27–28, 29, 99
nifedipine (Procardia, Adalat), 108, 182
nitrates, 125

Nitro-Dur (nitroglycerin), 108
nitrofurantoin, 83, 85
nitroglycerin (Nitro-Dur), 108
nonsteroidal anti-inflammatory drugs (NSAIDs): aspirin, 83, 135, 143, 146–151, 175; bleeding, 143, 145–151, 153–159, 157; hearing loss, 133, 135; ibuprofen, 46, 83, 159; kidney damage, 59, 60–65; naproxen, 67, 69, 70, 135, 153–159; pancreatitis, 83; Stevens-Johnson Syndrome, 187
Norco. *See* hydrocodone/acetaminophen
normeperidine, 3
Norpramin (desipramine), 107, 115
nortriptyline (Pamelor), 107, 115
Norvasc (amlodipine), 59–60, 61
Norvir (ritonavir), 115, 128
NSAIDs. *See* nonsteroidal anti-inflammatory drugs
Nubain (nalbuphine hydrochloride), 229
nursing homes, 208
Nyquil, 107

O
obesity, 174, 175
obsessive-complusive disorder (OCD) medications, 190–191
ofloxacin, 55
olmesartan, 49
omeprazole, 143, 151, 216
opioids/opiates: constipation, 164; drug names in category, 164; intestinal blockage, 161–166; respiratory insufficiency, 37–38, 40–42; withdrawals from, 224–230
OsCal 500, 66–72
osteoporosis medications, 151–159
ototoxicity, 130–135
overdoses, 42, 76–77, 221
oversight, lack of, 217–224
over-the-counter (OTC) medicines: adverse drug reaction awareness, 18, 72, 78–79, 159; adverse reaction recording and reporting, 23; antacids, 67–72; herbal products, 114, 115, 182; label directions and warnings, 71; laxatives, 33, 34–36, 165–166; pain medications

(*See* acetaminophen; nonsteroidal anti-inflammatory drugs); stool softeners, 162, 165
oxybutynin (Ditropan), 108
oxycodone (Oxycotin, OxyIR), 161–162, 163–166

P

Pacerone (amiodarone), 25–31, 56, 96, 128, 143
pain medications: constipation, 164; falling, 108; intestinal blockage, 161–162, 162–166; liver damage, 73–74; metaxalone, 199; respiratory insufficiency, 38–44; seizures, 3–4, 5, 122; serotonin syndrome, 115; tramadol, 80, 122; withdrawals from opiate, 225, 226–230. *See also* acetaminophen; hydrocodone/acetaminophen; nonsteroidal anti-inflammatory drugs
Pamelor (nortriptyline), 107, 115
pancreatitis, 79–84
pantoprazole, 151, 216
paranoid psychosis, 101
Parkinson's medications, 107, 108
Parlodel (bromocriptine), 108, 115
Parnate (tranylcypromine), 115, 191
paroxetine (Paxil), 115, 216
patient-year, defined, 142
Pedialyte, 210
penicillins, 187, 208
pentamidine, 56, 83
pentazocine, 229–230
pentazocine/naloxone, 230
pentobarbital (Nembutal), 108
Pepcid, 168
Percocet (acetaminophen and oxycodone), 230
perphenazine (Trilafon), 108, 216
phenelzine (Nardil), 43, 115, 191
phenobarbitals, 78, 187
phenytoin (Dilantin), 64, 78, 92–97, 117, 187, 216
pill boxes or planners, 143
pimozide, 56, 216
piroxicam, 135, 187
pneumonia, 31–36, 171

postmarketing surveillance, 7
potassium, 54, 198–204
PRAISE trial, 60
pravastatin, 194
prednisone (Sterapred, Deltasone), 99–103, 187
pregnancy, 32–33, 38, 46, 81, 85–86, 147, 152, 162
prescription compliance, 16, 71, 84–90, 158
PresTab (glyburide), 86–90, 108, 147
Prilosec, 71, 214
Prinivil (lisinopril), 32–34, 83, 108, 201
proactivity of patient, 8, 19–20, 223
Pro-Banthine (propantheline), 108
procainamide, 56, 121
Procardia (nifedipine), 108, 182
prochlorperazine (Compazine), 108, 211–215, 216
Prolixin, 108
promethazine, 216
propantheline (Pro-Banthine), 108
propranolol (Inderal), 108
Prosom (estazolam), 107
prostaglandins, 62
proton pump inhibitors (PPIs), 64, 71, 148–149, 151, 155, 216
protriptyline (Vivactil), 107, 115
Proventil (albuterol), 98–99
Prozac (fluoxetine), 115, 230
psychosis, 91–97, 98–103
psychotropics, 56, 108

Q

QTc intervals, 57
quinapril (Accupril), 45–46, 108
quinidine, 56, 128
quinine, 135
quinolones, 52, 53–57, 143, 187, 208

R

ramipril, 45–46, 118, 199–204
ranitidine (Zantac), 71
rasagiline (Azilect), 108, 191
rashes, 118, 181–189
reconciliation, 19–20, 217–220, 221–224
Reglan (metoclopramide), 108, 161, 211, 213–214, 216

Remeron (mirtazapine), 92
renal function. *See* kidney (renal) function
reporting, 2, 6–8, 23. *See also* MedWatch
Requip (ropinirole), 108
respiratory insufficiency, 37–44
Restoril (temazepam), 85–86, 107, 108
Revex (nalmefene hydrochloride), 230
Reye's syndrome, 146
rhabdomyolysis, 147, 189–198
rifampin, 64, 78
risedronate (Actonel), 155
risperidone (Risperdal), 108
Risperdal (risperidone), 108
ritonavir, 115, 128
Rolaids, 66–72
Romazicon (flumazenil), 221
ropinirole (Requip), 108
rotigotine (Neupro), 108
Roxanol (morphine), 108

S
salicylates, 135, 146. *See also* aspirin
schizophrenia, 101
scopolamine, 108
secobarbital (Seconal), 108
Seconal (secobarbital), 108
seizures, 3–4, 5, 116–122, 122, 182
selective serotonin reuptake inhibitors (SSRIs), 110–116, 121, 190–191, 230
self-dosing, 16, 71, 84–90, 158
senna, 165, 166
serotonin syndrome, 109–116, 191
sertraline (Zoloft), 115, 216, 230
serum creatinine (SCr), 14, 169, 172
Serzone (nefazodone), 115
shock, 150
simvastatin, 45, 67, 190–198
simvastatin/ezetimibe, 45, 67
Sinequan (doxepine), 107, 115, 216
6-mercaptopurine, 83
SJS (Stevens-Johnson Syndrome), 147, 181–189
Skelaxin (metaxalone), 108, 199
sleeping aids, 32, 34, 60, 85–86, 104–108
smoking, 25, 27–28, 29, 99
sodium deficiencies, 118–122

Soma, 104–107
sotalol, 56
sprironolactone, 198–199, 201–204
SSRIs (selective serotonin reuptake inhibitors), 110–116, 121, 190–191, 230
St. John's wort, 114, 115
Stadol NS, 226–230
statins, 147, 190–198
Stelazine (trifluoperazine), 108
Sterapred (prednisone), 99–103, 187
Stevens-Johnson Syndrome (SJS), 147, 181–189
stool softeners, 162
street drugs, 115
streptomycin, 135
Suboxone (buprenorphine and naloxone), 229
Subutex (buprenorphine), 229
suicide and suicidal ideation, 60, 93, 101, 110, 191
sulfa allergies, 124, 131, 137, 182
sulfamethoxazole/trimethoprim, 143, 182–187
sulfonamides, 83, 208
sulindac, 135
Symmetrel (amantadine), 115
Synthroid (levothyroxine), 111

T
tacrolimus, 64, 197
Tagamet (cimetidine), 71, 168, 170
Talwin (pentazocine and naloxone), 229–230
Talwin NX, 230
Tegretol/Tegretol XR. *See* carbamazepine
telmisartan (Micardis), 49, 81, 202
temazepam (Restoril), 85–86, 107, 108
TEN (toxic epidermal necrolysis), 185
Tenormin (atenolol), 108, 205
Tequin (gatifloxacin), 55
TESS (Toxic Exposure Surveillance System), 114
tetracyclines, 83, 208
theophylline, 122
thioridazine, 44, 56, 216
Thorazine (chlorpromazine), 56, 108, 122, 216

thyroid replacement therapies, 111
tobramycin, 135
Tofranil (imipramine), 107, 115
tolerance, 15–16
Toprol XL (metoprolol succinate), 26, 51
torsades de pointes (arrhythmia), 50–57
torsemide (Demadex), 108
toxic epidermal necrolysis (TEN), 185
Toxic Exposure Surveillance System
    (TESS), 114
tramadol, 80, 115, 122
tranquilizers, 56, 108
Tranxene (clorazepate), 107
tranylcypromine (Parnate), 115, 191
trazodone, 60, 63, 115
tremors, 210–216
triazolam, 107
Tricor (fenofibrate), 195, 197
trifluoperazine (Stelazine), 108
Trihexane (trihexyphenidyl), 108, 216
trihexyphenidyl (Trihexane, Artane),
    108, 216
Trilafon (perphenazine), 108, 216
trimethoprim/sulfamethoxazole, 143,
    182–187
tryptophan, 115
Tums, 66–72
Tylenol. See acetaminophen
Tylenol with Codeine, 108

U

ulcerations, gastrointestinal, 151–159
Ultram (tramadol), 80, 115, 122
Unithroid (levothyroxine), 111
Univasc (moexipril), 45–46, 201, 202
urinary incontinence medications, 107,
    108

V

Valium (diazepam), 107, 199, 219–224,
    230

valproate, 216
valproic acid (Depakene/Depakote), 83,
    96, 108, 120, 187
valsartan (Diovan), 49, 81, 202
Vaseretic (enalapril and hydrochlorothia-
    zide), 152, 201
Vasotec (enalapril), 45–46, 83, 108, 152
venlafaxine, 115
Ventolin (albuterol), 98–99
verapamil (Verelan, Calan), 108, 128
Verelan (verapamil), 108, 128
Vicodin. See hydrocodone/acetamino-
    phen
Vistaril (hydroxyzine), 107
vitamins, 36, 141, 143, 153
Vivactil (protriptyline), 107, 115
Vivitrol (naltrexone), 230
vomiting, 146, 148, 151, 157–158, 165, 211
Vytorin (ezetimibe and simvastatin), 45,
    67

W

warfarin, 13, 18, 36, 96, 136–145, 149, 182
Wellbutrin (bupropion), 115, 122
withdrawals, 224–230

X

Xanax (alprazolam), 107, 211, 230

Z

Zantac (ranitidine), 71
Zarontin (ethosuximide), 96, 108
Zaroxolyn (metolazone), 108
Zestril (lisinopril), 32–34, 83, 108, 201
Zetia (ezetimibe), 67, 205
Zocor (simvastatin), 45, 67, 190–198
Zoloft (sertraline), 115, 216, 230
zolpidem, 104–105
Zyloprim (allopurinol), 64, 187
Zyvox (linezolid), 115